Burk Jubelt, M.D.
Department of Neurology
Suny Health Science Center
Syracuse, New York 13210

Burk Jubelt, M.D
Department of Neurology
Suny Health Science Center
Syracuse, New York 13210

Chronic Fatigue
Syndrome

Burk Jubelt, M.D.
Department of Neurology
Suny Health Science Center
Syracuse, New York 13210

Chronic Fatigue Syndrome

Edited by

DAVID M. DAWSON, M.D.
Professor of Neurology, Harvard Medical School, Boston; Chief, Neurology Service, Brockton/West Roxbury Veterans Administration Medical Center, West Roxbury, Massachusetts

THOMAS D. SABIN, M.D.
Professor of Neurology and Psychiatry, Boston University School of Medicine; Director, Neurological Unit, Boston City Hospital, Boston

Little, Brown and Company
Boston/Toronto/London

Library of Congress Cataloging-in-Publication Data

Chronic fatigue syndrome / edited by David M. Dawson, Thomas D. Sabin.
    p. cm.
  Includes bibliographical references and index.
  ISBN 0-316-17748-2 (cloth)
  1. Chronic fatigue syndrome. I. Dawson, D. M. (David Michael),
1930–   . II. Sabin, Thomas D.
  [DNLM: 1. Fatigue Syndrome, Chronic. WL 351 C557]
RB150.F37C47 1993
616'.047—dc20
DNLM/DLC
for Library of Congress   92-49249
                                                    CIP

Printed in the United States of America

RRD-VA

Sponsoring Editor: Nancy Chorpenning
Production Editor: Kellie Cardone
Copyeditor: Nancy Megley
Indexer: Julia Figures
Production Supervisor: F. David Bell
Designer: F. David Bell
Cover Designer: Linda Dana Willis

Burk Jubelt, M.D.
Department of Neurology
Suny Health Science Center
Syracuse, New York 13210

Contents

Contributing Authors

Peter O. Behan, Ch.B., M.D., F.R.C.P. (L) (G) (I)
Professor of Neurology, University of Glasgow; Department of
Neurology, Institute of Neurological Sciences, Southern General
Hospital, Glasgow, Scotland

Wilhelmina M. H. Behan, M.D., F.R.C.P.
Senior Lecturer in Pathology, University of Glasgow; Honorary
Consultant in Pathology, Western Infirmary, Glasgow, Scotland

Heather M. A. Cavanagh, Ph.D.
Senior Research Fellow, Department of Neurology, University of
Glasgow, Southern General Hospital, Glasgow, Scotland

Grace Chang, M.D., M.P.H.
Instructor of Psychiatry, Harvard Medical School; Attending
Psychiatrist, Brigham and Women's Hospital, Boston

David M. Dawson, M.D.
Professor of Neurology, Harvard Medical School, Boston; Chief,
Neurology Service, Brockton/West Roxbury Veterans Administration
Medical Center, West Roxbury, Massachusetts

Ian Downie, M.Sc., B.Sc.
Research Assistant, Department of Pathology, Western Infirmary,
Glasgow, Scotland

Nelson Gantz, M.D.
Clinical Professor of Medicine, Pennsylvania State University College
of Medicine, Hershey; Chief, Division of Infectious Diseases, and
Chairman, Department of Medicine, Polyclinic Medical Center,
Harrisburg, Pennsylvania

Don L. Goldenberg, M.D.
Professor of Medicine, Tufts University School of Medicine, Boston;
Chief of Rheumatology, Newton-Wellesley Hospital, Newton,
Massachusetts

John W. Gow, Ph.D.
Lecturer, Neurology Department, Southern General Hospital,
Glasgow, Scotland

Anthony L. Komaroff, M.D.
Associate Professor of Medicine, Harvard Medical School; Director,
Division of General Medicine, Brigham and Women's Hospital,
Boston

Robert G. Miller, M.D.
Clinical Professor of Neurology, University of California, San
Francisco, School of Medicine; Neurologist in Chief, California Pacific
Medical Center, San Francisco

Harvey Moldofsky, M.D.
Professor of Psychiatry and Medicine, University of Toronto Faculty of
Medicine; Director, Centre for Sleep and Chronobiology, Toronto
Western Division, The Toronto Hospital, Toronto

Ian A. R. More, Ph.D., M.D., F.R.C.P.
Senior Lecturer, Department of Pathology, University of Glasgow;
Consultant, Department of Pathology, Western Infirmary, Glasgow,
Scotland

Lindsay J. A. Morrison, Ph.D.
Lecturer, Department of Neurology, University of Glasgow; Institute
of Neurological Sciences, Southern General Hospital, Glasgow,
Scotland

Louis Reik, Jr., M.D.
Associate Professor of Neurology, University of Connecticut School of
Medicine, University of Connecticut Health Center; Attending
Neurologist, John Dempsey Hospital, Farmington, Connecticut

Malcolm P. Rogers, M.D.
Assistant Professor of Psychiatry, Harvard Medical School; Director of
Ambulatory Services, Psychiatry Division, Brigham and Women's
Hospital, Boston

Loren A. Rolak, M.D.
Associate Professor of Clinical Neurology, Baylor College of Medicine;
Assistant Chief of Neurology, Veterans Administration Medical
Center, Houston

Thomas D. Sabin, M.D.
Professor of Neurology and Psychiatry, Boston University School of
Medicine; Director, Neurological Unit, Boston City Hospital, Boston

Richard B. Schwartz, M.D., Ph.D.
Assistant Professor of Radiology, Harvard Medical School; Assistant
Director of Neuroradiology, Department of Radiology, Brigham and
Women's Hospital, Boston

Kathleen Simpson, B.Sc.
Research Assistant, Department of Neurology, University of Glasgow,
Southern General Hospital, Glasgow, Scotland

Lewis Sudarsky, M.D.
Assistant Professor of Neurology, Harvard Medical School, Boston;
Assistant Chief of Neurology, Brockton/West Roxbury Veterans
Administration Medical Center, West Roxbury, Massachusetts

Thomas R. Swift, M.D.
Professor and Chairman, Department of Neurology, Medical College
of Georgia School of Medicine, Augusta, Georgia

Preface

This book covers a controversial topic. Most texts or monographs are written when the subjects they discuss have reached a certain level of development, and workers in the field share and agree on a certain body of knowledge.

The chronic fatigue syndromes have not reached that status. As we will show, similar illnesses have been described before, often in epidemics. Various names have been proposed, including epidemic neuromyasthenia, Iceland disease, Royal Free disease, and myalgic encephalomyelitis. Some of these names persist; their number is a measure of lack of consensus. In the United States, following a surge of interest and several recent publications, the term *chronic fatigue syndrome* (CFS) has gained wide acceptance. Diagnostic criteria have been proposed, and a number of conferences of workers in the field have been convened. Nevertheless, there is little unanimity about the existence of CFS or, if it exists, what its cause might be.

We have edited this volume from the point of view of clinical neurologists. Neither of us has been exposed to an epidemic of CFS. Each has seen, over the course of many years of clinical experience in different settings, patients who seem to fit into this category of illness. We believe other neurologists have seen such patients, too, although the reactions of physicians to patients with these kinds of complaints vary widely. Some deny that they exist; others are skeptical; still others are frustrated by the lack of clear diagnostic or therapeutic guidelines.

This volume presents the available information about the clinical syndrome. We have tried to open up discussion of neurologic issues: hence the chapters by Miller, by Moldofsky, and by Sudarsky about possible mechanisms of fatigue in the central nervous system and how they may be measured. Crucial psychiatric aspects of CFS are covered by Rogers and Chang. The role of neuroimaging in the diagnosis and understanding of CFS as well as the relationship to the MRI of demyelinating disease is presented by Schwartz. Chapters by Gantz, Behan, Komaroff, and Goldenberg set forth the views of physicians who have seen many patients and who approach the matter from the perspective of an internist, rheumatologist, or immunologist. Chapters by Reik, Rolak, and Swift present information on other neurologic illnesses sometimes confounded with or overlapping with CFS.

A continuing mystery is the nature of the epidemics that sweep through population groups from time to time. Some aspects of these outbreaks suggest transmissibility. What has been transmitted? Evidence of a viral cause of CFS has remained evanescent, although Behan and his co-workers—long-time proponents of a viral cause—present evidence indicating persistence of a viral genome.

Clearly, speculation about CFS will continue. Disabled patients continue to need care. Committed lay groups as well as concerned professionals have a long way to go. We hope we show some current directions.

D. M. D.
T. D. S.

Chronic Fatigue Syndrome

NOTICE

The indications and dosages of all drugs in this book have been recommended in the medical literature and conform to the practices of the general medical community. The medications described do not necessarily have specific approval by the Food and Drug Administration for use in the diseases and dosages for which they are recommended. The package insert for each drug should be consulted for use and dosage as approved by the FDA. Because standards for usage change, it is advisable to keep abreast of revised recommendations, particularly those concerning new drugs.

1

Thomas D. Sabin
David M. Dawson

History and Epidemiology

The fatigue pains that arise in the body are as follow. Men out of training suffer these pains after the slightest exercise, as no part of their body has been inured to any exercise; but trained bodies feel fatigue pains after unusual exercises, some even after usual exercises if they be excessive. These are the various kinds of fatigue pains; their properties are as follow. Untrained people, whose flesh is moist, after exercise undergo a considerable melting as the body grows warm. Now whatever of this melted substance passes out as sweat, or is purged away with the breath, causes pain only to the part of the body that has been emptied contrary to custom; but such part of it as remains behind causes pain not only to the part of the body emptied contrary to custom, but also to the part that has received the moisture as it is not congenial to the body but hostile to it.

Hippocrates[1]

Hippocrates at least recognized the muscular fatigue of deconditioning. The more modern beginnings of the concept of clinically significant fatigue trace back to eighteenth century mechanistic notions regarding nervous energy [2,3]. The nervous "machine" could be overenergized and develop an "irritability" that was associated with mental illness. Alternatively, the amount of energy available in the machine could be run down, and from this notion the original idea of neurasthenia came into existence. George Miller Beard popularized the idea that nervous energy becomes exhausted in his 1869 article, and coined the term *neurasthenia* [4]. The idea was taken up with considerable enthusiasm by an American founder of neurology, S. Weir Mitchell, who became a vocal advocate of his "rest cure" required to restore the energy of the nervous system and heal neurasthenia in these patients [5]. Every era since has had its fad involving a vague diagnostic entity for sufferers of chronic fatigue. The recent epidemics of postviral fatigue have provided the most important, but not unalloyed, evidence for the existence of a specific medical entity.

If there is in the universe an opposite for all things, then surely the epidemics of tarantism serve this role for epidemic fatigue. In these bizarre epidemics, entire villages would take to dancing in the streets with hilarious ravings. The marked overactivity ultimately resulted in profound exhaustion and sometimes ended fatally: Some sufferers bashed in their skulls or leaped to a watery death.

These events may have been due to ergotism, but at the time they posed the same dilemma between a psychosocial model and a medical model that the chronic fatigue syndrome (CFS) does today. Who would have believed then that fatal insomnia was a transmissible familial prion disorder [6]? Zinsser pointed out that while many of the episodes of tarantism may have been simply mass hysteria in response to the horrors of unremitting war, famine, and repetitive visits from the Black Plague, some patients were recurrently affected with bouts of hyperactivity and others had residual tremors after the acute form of the illness [7]. Zinsser concluded:

> . . . in great part no doubt the outbreaks were hysterical reactions of the terror stricken and wretched population which had broken down under the stress of an almost incredible hardship and danger. But it seems likely that associated with these were nervous diseases of infectious origin which followed the great epidemics and plagues, smallpox, etc., in the same manner in which neurotropic virus diseases have followed the widespread and severe epidemics which accompanied the last war.

This commentary was written in 1934, the same year in which the first epidemic of CFS was reported. That report, from Los Angeles, did not put the syndrome on the map, however. It was not until the 1948 outbreak in Iceland that widespread interest in the problem was renewed.

THE EPIDEMICS

Los Angeles, 1934

Coincident with a polio epidemic in 1934, 198 employees of the Los Angeles County General Hospital were affected with a disease that was at first thought to be polio [8]. Many individuals were part of the team caring for the patients with polio. The attack rate of the "new" disease was very high in the population at risk: 4.4% of all hospital employees were affected, and attack rates of 10.7% among the nurses and 5.4% of the physicians were observed. During this time, more than 2000 cases of polio were occurring in Los Angeles County.

The nonpolio illness did not have the sharp onset of fever and meningeal symptoms soon giving way to persistent and definitely localized flaccid weakness that characterized true poliomyelitis. Another feature that separated these patients from the polio patients was a tendency for recurrence, often with gradually increasing disability. Motor findings were late in onset and no atrophy was noted. Two patients were placed on respirators. Sensory complaints were much more frequent than in polio. Muscle tenderness occurred, often associated with twitching that at times amounted to actual muscle spasms. Intense fatigue, personality change, irritability and depression, insomnia, and difficulty with memory and concentration all emerged as prominent and persistent features in these patients but not in the polio patients. One physician had ". . . repeated emotional upsets for no apparent cause and developed violent dislikes for people and things formerly liked." Spells of depression and outbursts of weeping for no apparent cause were also mentioned. Some autonomic difficulties such as limb edema and sweating without fever were also noted. Twelve percent of the patients had inability to urinate that required catheterization.

Laboratory analysis in these cases was limited, but 59 lumbar punctures were performed. Pleocytosis was noted in three patients with cell counts of 12 to 66 lymphocytes. The search for abnormal globulins at that time was limited to the colloidal gold precipitation test, which was abnormal in 18 of the 59 patients who had lumbar puncture. The cerebrospinal fluid (CSF) pressures recorded in these patients were often slightly elevated.

Pooled human serum injections were widely used as polio prophylaxis during this era as a means of creating immunity among those working with the disease. This factor may have modified a polio infection or had a role in inducing another disorder.

Patient contacts in this epidemic were looked at closely, and personal contact appeared to be the most likely mode of transmission. The residential nursing staff working in the polio wards and in the admitting office were affected first, followed by student and graduate nurses not living on the hospital grounds, and then students and graduates who were not working in the communicable disease wards; the last affected group were nonresident graduate nurses working on the nonpolio wards. Gilliam concluded his detailed analysis of the spread of this illness with the suggestion of spread by personal contact and indicated "good grounds for assuming that the majority of them resulted from an infection with the virus of poliomyelitis." He also commented that "certain observers were of the privately expressed opinion that hysteria played a large role in this outbreak. While it cannot be denied that hysteria was an important factor in some cases it appears extremely unlikely that many of the cases were purely hysterical in nature."

Iceland, 1948

Akureyri, a town of 6900 residents on the northern coast of Iceland, was the focus of an important epidemic in the early winter of 1948–49 [9]. Within the township, 488 cases occurred within 3 months with an incidence of 6.7% in the town itself and 0.8% in the rural districts around the town. This epidemic was not focused on medical personnel but once again was initially misdiagnosed as poliomyelitis. The sparing of young children, prominence of sensory symptoms, and prolongation into chronicity clinically separated this disease from polio. The illness spread to other districts in Iceland, and in at least one instance sequential cases were recorded along the land route from Akureyri to Reykjavik.

The demographic characteristics of Iceland made epidemiologic studies quite precise. While young children were generally spared, the highest attack rates were in the 15- to 19-year age group. Clusters in high schools and in homes were the rule. One boarding home for high school students had 29 of its 49 residents affected. Females were more often affected than males, and the analysis of contacts was consistent with an incubation of 5 to 8 days.

The illness typically began with pain in the neck and shoulders and a mild fever. Onset could be acute or subacute. Paresthesias and muscle tenderness were very prominent. The tenderness could be quite conspicuous and at times was confined to "small spots in the muscle" (of interest in relation to fibromyalgia; see Chapter 5). Burning, aching sensations were present in one or more limbs with tiredness out of proportion to other aspects of the illness. Sensory loss was sometimes not anatomically distributed; at other times it was thought to be in specific segmental or peripheral nerve distributions. In paralytic cases, muscle twitching was often present for 3 to 7 days before weakness ensued. The weakness was often associated with physical exertion or exposure to cold and was anticipated by an associated increase in local pain. Atrophy was noted but was rare. Except for a single case involving the tongue, the motor and cranial nerves were spared and retention of deep tendon reflexes was the rule. No patients had extensor plantar responses. There was a scattering of autonomic dysfunction with urine retention occurring in two patients, and abnormal patterns of sweating, constipation, and palpitations were recorded. Many patients complained of persistent tiredness, nervousness, and insomnia.

Long-term follow-up was available for this epidemic. The first review was 7 to 10 months after the original epidemic and involved assessment of 57 patients [9]. It was not clear how this group was chosen, but only 11% thought they had fully recovered. The others complained of persistent nervousness, tiredness, pains often in a definite radicular distribution, postexertional tiredness in previously paretic limbs, insomnia, and difficulty with memory. About one third of the patients continued to have muscle tenderness and one fourth had muscle weakness and atrophy. Seventeen percent were considered to have hysterical paresis and 14% hysterical sensory disturbances. The authors expressed concern about the possibility of a hysterical illness and stated [9]:

. . . during an epidemic of this magnitude and nature it is to be expected that hysterical symptoms be observed either alone or in conjunction with genuine symptoms of the epidemic disease. This has throughout been very much in our minds, but we feel that the *clinical* picture as presented here is not grossly distorted or confused by such symptoms or complaints. It is conceivable, however, that a sufficient number of functional disorders may have occurred to influence to some extent the number of reported cases and the sex distribution of this epidemic.

Pleocytosis and elevated spinal fluid protein were seen in a few patients, but no other significant laboratory data were recorded despite extensive search for bacteriologic and virologic agents. There was also no evidence of contamination of the milk or water supply.

Six years after the Akureyri outbreak 39 of the original patients, 33 females and 6 males, were reassessed [10]. All but one (who had a gastric ulcer) were back at work, but only 13% considered themselves recovered and 69% had objective clinical signs. The most common complaint was nervousness and general tiredness, but muscle pain, sleeplessness, and memory difficulty were all noted. The authors indicated that "in 1949 several of the patients were neurotic and showed functional symptoms. This was still the case in June 1955 but only those symptoms which seemed to be organic had been included in the Tables."

Yet another follow-up was completed 40 years later [11]. This involved nine patients from the 1948 epidemic and one affected in 1955. The authors noted that three of the ten patients had had a 2-week episode in 1947—the year before their chronic illness—characterized by burning limb pain, prostration, and muscle weakness. One of these patients was the physical education teacher at the high school, which had a high incidence of disease during the epidemic. One of the 10 patients mentioned recurrences after the initial few years, and eight indicated that they never fully recovered. The authors noted no obvious hysteria or neuroticism in these patients nor was there a suggestion of depression, although two patients admitted that they had experienced severe depressions earlier in the disease. Two women who originally experienced severe paralysis had functionally recovered although they had persistent muscle weakness. All these patients still reported general fatigue, muscle pain, tenderness, weakness, and numbness, and also complained that many in the medical profession considered them to be "hysterical."

Australia, 1949

In May 1949, an epidemic of poliomyelitis broke out in Adelaide [12, 13]. In August of that year it became clear that another epidemic was occurring contemporaneously with polio, initially recognized by lack of cells in the CSF of the atypical patients. Of 1350 patients admitted to the hospital, 800 had fewer than 10 cells per milliliter; only 10% or so of patients with polio would have been expected to have such a low CSF cell count. The actual number of patients with the acute nonpolio illness was not known.

Some patients had an insidious onset with symptoms of being "off color" for several months. Most began with malaise and severe headache. Stiff neck and back were constant. Muscle pain persisted in almost every patient for up to 6 months, but weakness was slight. The behavioral phenomena that complicated this disease were consistent and the cause of greatest disability. Inability to concentrate and depression were the most common symptoms. Overall the prognosis was good, even for the psychologic disturbances, which eventually resolved. Pellew remarked that "reassurance backed by tonics worked best" [12]. In 1955, laboratory investigations were reported for five patients who had been further studied. Two of five monkeys inoculated with patients' mixed feces, CSF, and throat washings developed an inflammatory radiculopathy in the lumbosacral roots [13].

New York State, 1950

This outbreak in the late summer and early fall of 1950 was not well documented from the epidemiologic standpoint. The 19 patients analyzed were simply drawn from the practice of one of the authors [14]. No personal contact with another case was documented for 10 of the 19 individuals. Again, polio was prevalent in the community at the time, and the authors noted that many cases in the region diagnosed as "abortive polio" or "polio suspect" may have actually been this "other illness."

The major differences from polio were the intensity and persistence of the muscle aching, which was associated with marked tenderness especially around the shoulders but also involving arms, neck, back, and lower extremities. There was also chest pain worsened by breathing but without actual pleurisy. Hyperesthesia of the skin overlying the sore muscles often was present, but weakness did not necessarily involve the tender muscles. The weakness was once again incomplete and not associated with atrophy. Deep tendon reflexes were either normal or transiently depressed. One of the patients (with 27 white cells per microliter in his spinal fluid) had ". . . one small localized spot on the left. This was extremely tender and gave a sensation of crepitus to the palpating fingers when the muscle fibers were moved against the edge of the scapula"—yet another account of a finding associated with fibromyalgia (see Chapter 5). The authors also pointed out the prominence of severe depressive states with bouts of crying for no apparent reason, even among patients previously described as quite stoic.

The fluctuating nature of the symptoms and vagueness of the objective findings led these authors as well to express their concern about the possibility of a functional illness. They commented [14]:

The common incidence of mental depression, vagueness of many of the symptoms, and absence of objective physical signs must of course raise the question whether this is a distinct disease entity or whether it is a non-specific fever in neurotic and suggestible patients. This possibility was prominent in our minds from the beginning but we became quite convinced that this clinical syndrome could not be explained away as a neurotic reaction to a fever. Other symptoms and signs of neurosis were not found and the group examined had in the past shown no higher incidence of neurotic illness than is ordinarily found in the general population.

The onset in these cases was similar to that in the other epidemics, with headache, muscle aching, sore throat, respiratory and gastrointestinal distress, and low-grade fevers. Lymphadenopathy occurred in four patients and weakness without true wasting was noted in 13 of the 19. Paresthesias and numbness often showed no definite anatomic pattern, although one patient was said to have lost joint position in the lower extremities for 2 weeks. Laboratory evaluations showed only one other patient with transient appearance of white blood cells in the spinal fluid, though protein was normal. Some of the patients had elevated urinary creatine excretion. The authors noted the similarity to the Iceland outbreak.

Follow-up was possible for 8 of the 19 patients 15 months after the original illness, and none of them felt normal. Most complained of tiring easily with muscle aching brought on by minimal exertion and "damp weather." Seven of the 8 continued to have emotional abnormalities, particularly depression or anxiety. Tenderness of the muscles, weakness, and sensory loss were found at follow-up in the same distribution as was noted early in the course of the illness.

London (Middlesex Hospital), 1952

Between July and September 1952, 14 nurses residing at the Middlesex Hospital were affected. Seven of the cases occurred in August [15]. The illness can be compared with, and possibly associated with, outbreaks in Berlin in November 1954 (among British soldiers stationed there), two cases reported by Sumner that occurred in 1955 [16], a group of cases reported from the referral area near Coventry from 1953 [17], further scattered cases from Coventry from 1956 [18], patients with encephalomyelitis simulating poliomyelitis from London in 1955 [19, 20], and finally the large epidemic at the Royal Free Hospital in 1955 [21] that contributed one of the many names for this illness, "Royal Free disease" described later in the chapter. It may be that all these epidemics in England during the 1950s were related, or it may be that awareness of the illness was high among area practitioners at the time.

Denmark, 1952

The diagnosis of "vegetative neuritis" was used to describe a number of patients in Denmark who suffered from an illness characterized by severe fatigue, relapses, and autonomic symptoms [22]. The epidemic once again occurred while there was polio in the community, and 3 of the 10 patients described had definite exposure to poliomyelitis; 4 of the 10 were actually hospital employees. The 10 patients described in detail in the available reference happened to be referred to the author for his evaluation, and therefore information about the epidemiology or case prevalence during this period is not known. All 10 patients were young women between the ages of 20 and 40.

The onset was fairly acute with headache and neckache accompanied by nausea, vomiting, and dizziness or wooziness. There were also strange paresthesias, often with sensations of coldness, which did not follow root or peripheral nerve distributions. Paresthesias affected the face around the lips or in the cheeks and would sometimes migrate from one limb to another. Although the patients complained of weakness, paralysis was seen in only one, and in that patient no signs of anterior horn cell destruction were found. Marked tenderness over muscles was again seen. Low-grade fevers or irregularity in the temperature curves were also described. One patient was acutely sensitive to noise. Patients often had abnormalities in their pattern of sweating or persistent vasoconstriction in the extremities. There were frequent behavioral changes. All felt tired. One patient was unable to read because she fatigued with mental concentration. Others became fearful, irritable, or impatient as well as being depressed. The spinal fluid was examined in 5 of the 10 patients and was unrevealing.

Bethesda, 1953

This epidemic involved a total of 50 patients [23]. Early summer was the season, and young adults, but not children, were once more the patients. Thirty-nine patients were nurses or student nurses, and although it was polio season, these nurses were involved instead in the care of psychiatric patients. One of the unique epidemiologic features of this episode was that 2 ½ months after the first group of cases, a second small cluster appeared among a group of students newly arrived at the institution for their psychiatry rotation.

All of the patients shared common environmental features although the hospital was a campus-type institution with multiple buildings. Analysis of contact patterns suggested an incubation period of 5 to 8 days. Analyses of food, dairy products, water and ice, the swimming pond, insect vectors, and a search for toxins were all unrevealing. There was no large-scale involvement in the community surrounding the hospital, nor were there any cases in the schools of origin for the student nurses doing this one affiliation at the affected psychiatric hospital. Further-more, no cases occurred among the husbands or boyfriends of the affected nurses! All this suggested some shared environmental factor rather than person-to-person transmission as a source of the disorder. While the nurses were in contact with each other, they were very likely in closer contact with patients, but among the patients there was only one questionable case.

The possibility of a psychiatric factor also lurked in the minds of observers of this outbreak, and they stated: "to decrease the possibility of including patients whose symptoms resulted from anxiety and apprehension but may have simulated the minor illness our description of the clinical manifestations is limited to the records of the 26 confirmed paretic cases." The definition of a paretic case included patients whose muscle weakness was recorded by at least two observers as abnormal and further confirmed by quantitative muscle testing procedures done at the biophysics research laboratory in Bethesda. The paralyses were distinctly unusual, weakness tending to occur 4 to 6 days after the onset. Heaviness and numbness in the limbs often preceded paresis. The strength declined only to 50 to 75% of normal, and again the deep tendon reflexes remained normal and there was no atrophy or flaccidity. Twenty-six of the 50 cases were classified as paretic.

Clinical features during the acute phase consisted of intense muscle aches and pains, particularly at the insertion of the diaphragm along the chest wall where "bands of pain" were experienced. Among the 26 paretic patients, both legs were weak in 25 and one arm was weak in 16. The leg weakness was symmetric but the upper extremity weakness mostly occurred in the right arm and hand. The patients complained of neck and back stiffness without actual signs of meningismus. There was headache, often made more severe by sitting up but not related to lumbar puncture. Diarrhea, temperature instability, and severe prostration with fatigability completed the picture. The authors commented that to look at the temperature heights was not particularly impressive as they usually did not go above 100.4°F (38°C), but there were marked temperature swings, sometimes 2 to 3°F each day. Other possible autonomic disturbances included rapid changes in skin color and moisture, limb edema, urinary frequency, and anorexia. Sensory changes were described as "nonsegmental" with either increased or decreased thresholds on testing to the usual modalities. Unprovoked crying spells, inability for sustained mental concentration, undue irritability, and increased anxiety were also mentioned in this epidemic as well as rarer instances of menstrual irregularities, anorexia, insomnia, and rarely local myoclonus and tremors. Follow-up is limited, but reexamination of 12 patients several months later revealed that none had returned to normal. Those able to work were doing so with great difficulty, sometimes only part-time, and most required bed rest during the day.

Twenty-five lumbar punctures were performed; there were always fewer than 5 lymphocytes, and three patients showed mild elevations of CSF protein to 48, 58, and 61 mg/dl. State-of-the-art virologic studies at that time were not revealing, but 12 of the 38 nurses were excreting Bethesda-Ballerup paracolon bacilli of the *Citrobacter* group and positive agglutinins for these bacilli were present in 22 of 39 patients.

Addington Hospital (South Africa), 1955

A rather remarkable outbreak of our "mystery illness" followed a polio epidemic in South Africa in February 1955 [24]. The initial report was of 84 nurses from a nurses' residence associated with the Addington Hospital. Even more remarkable was the fact that the illness apparently struck only persons of European extraction and did not affect either ward patients at the hospital or children.

The acute illness began with headache, extreme lassitude, sore throat, sore eyes, nausea, vomiting, diarrhea, backache, and coryza. During the acute phase, patients often complained of sudden weakness and heaviness in one or more extremities. The left side was more involved than the right. This was associated with pain in the muscles of the shoulder girdle, subcostal region, and low back as well as cramps in the affected muscles. There was no bulbar involvement and no true neck rigidity. Some patients were noted to have mild facial weakness, and they had tenderness of groups of muscles or single muscles. These muscles had a firm, "rubbery" consistency on examination and the tone varied from hypotonic to hypertonic.

Several of the detailed descriptions would be compatible with functional diagnoses. For example, it was stated that "when tested against resistance the muscles contracted in a curious, interrupted or clonic fashion" [25]. A male patient is described with ". . . clonic-like features in that contraction of his arm against resistance results in a spread of the involuntary movements to the rest of the body, sustained for some length of time. The picture was very bizarre and almost like hysteria." No wasting or atrophy was found in follow-up of the patients. The deep tendon reflexes appeared to be depressed early on but were never abolished. A remarkable number of relapses occurred in these patients, and personality changes such as euphoria, depression, and sleeplessness were noted.

This epidemic, like the one in Punta Gorda (described later), raises the question of genetic susceptibility to the illness since blacks were apparently spared in both areas of the world. Others use these observations to support the notion of a culturally induced epidemic hysteria. The bizarre findings on motor and sensory examination were in keeping with a psychologic or nonorganic source.

Royal Free Hospital (London), 1955

In less than 2 weeks in July 1955, more than 70 members of the staff of the Royal Free Hospital in London were admitted for an acute illness that began with headache, sore throat, malaise, lassitude, vertigo, and limb pains [21]. The hospital had to be closed, and within 4 months 292 staff members had been stricken by this strange malady. Although the beds of the hospital were full during this period, only 12 inpatients were affected. In a retrospective on this disease, Ramsay noted that in sporadic cases and smaller epidemics, sedentary individuals were rarely affected, suggesting that inpatients were protected by inactivity [26]. Close study of the contact history indicated that the incubation period was 5 to 7 days. Since this hospital consisted of nine buildings scattered over several blocks in northwest London, it was an excellent opportunity for analysis of spread by personal contact [27].

While the presenting symptoms were not very different from those of many viral illnesses, the intensity of the malaise from the outset was the striking feature of this outbreak. Neck, back, and limb pain, which appeared at the onset or several weeks later on, was often intense and disproportionate to the systemic symptoms. Patients often complained of unsteadiness with rapid postural changes and occasionally suffered actual vertigo.

General examination revealed low-grade fevers, usually less than 37.4°C, associated with pharyngeal injection and tender, swollen lymph nodes, especially in the posterior cervical group. This feature had not been noted in prior epidemics.

The neurologic features were striking: 74% of the patients showed "objective evidence of an affection of the nervous system." Asymmetric pupil size and palsies of the third, sixth, and seventh cranial nerves were seen. Two patients had swallowing difficulty that required tube feedings, while another nine had severe bulbar palsies.

Other motor findings included weakness in segmental distribution associated with fasciculations but without other clinical or electrophysiologic evidence of chronic denervation. Hemiplegic patterns of weakness were also common, but the extensor plantar response was rare and spasticity did not develop. More often hypotonia was noted, but active or passive movement of affected limbs frequently resulted in prolonged, painful muscle spasms. The spasms often arose in limbs where sensory change had occurred yet tendon jerks were preserved. Attempted movement of an affected limb might also result in gross jerky movement of that limb, and this was deemed one of the most distinctive features of the epidemic. Occasional patients also showed more typical myoclonic jerks, but none had cerebellar ataxia. Three patients required crutches or braces for ambulation. In an era when polio was still common, these motor findings caused considerable difficulty with diagnosis.

Cutaneous sensory abnormalities appeared to be more frequent than involvement of deep sensation and tended to be present in the regions of most prominent motor deficit. Myelopathic syndromes with paraparesis and sensory loss as well as bladder difficulty occurred in about one fourth of the hospitalized patients. Personality changes were also prominent. There was a high incidence of panic attacks, nightmares, and severe depression. Some patients showed unrelenting crying while others showed excessive sleepiness. One retrospective look at this epidemic analyzed the neurologic symptoms and signs to marshal a case for epidemic hysteria [28]. The spinal fluid was always normal, and the electrophysiologic studies of that era were unrevealing.

Two patients died of unrelated causes. Examination of the nervous system in the first showed "no abnormality except for that attributable to either the septicemia or carcinomatosis" that had been the cause of death. The second patient was a 32-year-old woman who died of a sedative overdose 7 months after becoming ill. Clinically she was thought to have multiple sclerosis (MS). It was not clear whether the onset of that disease antedated the epidemic. Nevertheless, she had lesions compatible with MS in the hemispheres, cord, and brainstem. In addition, one section of the hypothalamus showed intense perivascular cuffing. This case has significance not only because of the prominence of fatigue seen in many MS patients, but also in view of the possible hypothalamic involvement in CFS.

Ramsay, in 1978, reviewed the records of 53 patients with the same malady admitted to the Royal Free Hospital between April 1955 and September 1957, and asserted that they provided further evidence for endemicity of the disease in this region of England [26]. Of these patients, only 13 were members of hospital staff. He also underscored the clinical evidence for autonomic dysfunction, since many of these individuals suffered orthostatic tachycardia, hypothermia, and irregularities of cutaneous circulatory control. He noted that paresis occurred in 67% of the patients but thought the terms did not accurately define the unusual form of muscle fatigability that was the dominant clinical feature of the disease and was distinct from any usual type of neurologic weakness. Long-term follow-up indicated that while there were patients who completely recovered, others showed no recovery at all, and yet another group were prone to relapses usually precipitated by physical exertion. Intervals between relapses could be as long as 4 years.

Punta Gorda, Florida, 1956

In the spring of 1956, the small community of Punta Gorda, Florida, population 2500, suffered an illness with fatigue as the major disabling symptom that had an attack rate calculated at 6.3% [29]. The fatigue was intense, prolonged, and debilitating. The other symptoms—now familiar—were headache, stiff neck, nausea, vomiting, and aching muscle pains. There were some menstrual irregularities and frequently marked emotional alterations including increased anxiety, memory problems, depression, and episodic crying that occurred without apparent provocation. Hyperventilation attacks and terrifying dreams were also described. Other patients had paresthesias, difficulty swallowing, vertigo, and double vision. After the acute illness, fatigue and associated "tension" or depression were the major disabling symptoms. Young and middle-aged adults were affected and there were no deaths. More females than males were hospitalized. Thirty cases came to the attention of the medical community. Of these patients, 21 were studied in detail and all were white, although 45% of the Punta Gorda population was black! A house-to-house survey yielded another 51 cases. There was a very high proportion of affected medical personnel (42%).

Unlike the Royal Free Hospital epidemic, sore throat and lymphadenopathy were not prominent and objective findings on physical examination were minimal. Twelve of the 21 intensively studied patients had impairment of touch, pain, and temperature, but the deficits were described as somewhat bizarre and did not conform to the usual distribution of nerve roots or peripheral nerves. Focal muscle tenderness, particularly in the trapezius, gastrocnemius, deltoid, forearm, and paraspinal muscles, was described in some patients, which again highlights this feature now associated with the fibromyalgia syndrome. Several patients complained of weakness but had completely normal neurologic examinations. A careful but unrevealing search was conducted for some common factor in the water supply, milk, food, cosmetics, soaps, insecticides, swimming sites, and arthropod vectors. Laboratory assessment of the patients failed to define a cause. Spinal fluid was examined in five patients. No lymphocytes were found in two and from three to six cells in the others, with normal protein and glucose levels.

In common with the other epidemics, this outbreak showed again the high attack rate among medical personnel and the disease's ability to cause very prolonged incapacity. The other feature of interest was that this small community suffered an attack rate of 6.3% and it was possible to do an essentially complete house-to-house survey to establish firm data.

New York Convent, 1961

This epidemic affected 26 of 69 nuns in a rural convent in New York State [30]. Younger nuns were affected with greater frequency than older ones. The symptoms were again fatigue, anorexia, headache, nausea, and dizziness, with muscle aches in the limbs and along the costal margins, and also often with sensations of throat "tightness." Mood and behavior alterations with depression, emotional upsets, and unprovoked crying spells as well as difficulty in sustaining mental concentration were all common. Paralyses were scattered, sometimes transient and nonanatomic. In one patient with a hemiparesis, 31 lymphocytes were present in the spinal fluid. No atrophy or reflex change was described. Nonanatomic areas of numbness were present. Muscle twitching and involuntary movements were noted. One patient with choreiform movements of the limbs associated with facial and hand paresthesias was "thought to be hysterical." There were mild abnormalities in temperature regulation, but no adenopathy was noted. Two of the four patients who had lumbar punctures showed increased lymphocytes, and during the course of the illness several patients had increased urinary creatine secretion. The authors noted that "physicians unfamiliar with the peculiar characteristics of previous epidemics which resembled the one described here might easily dismiss these cases as hysteria."

Later Outbreaks

For reasons that we do not understand, epidemics of CFS, epidemic neuromyasthenia, or similar illnesses were not subsequently reported for more than 10 years. The medical literature—rarely quiet—was silent on this issue for the decade of the 1970s. Did all the patients vanish? Was there a change in medical perceptions? Did the patients all end up in psychiatric clinics with a diagnosis of occult depression?

An epidemic of comparable type may have occurred in New Zealand in the middle 1980s [31]. A lay patient-support organization grew up in that country in the following years. A publication from West Otago in 1984 described 28 patients, all but three of them younger than age 45, who had tiredness, headache, myalgias, and mood and sleep disturbances [32]. Nevertheless, the authors concluded after a literature survey that "we see no justification for calling this illness myalgic encephalomyelitis."

A number of patients came to the attention of the medical world in Australia as well, and were extensively investigated by Lloyd and colleagues [33]. These authors found changes in ratios of T-cell subsets as well as reduced in vivo and in vitro immune responsiveness in 100 patients compared with 100 controls. The same investigators also published data on the prevalence of CFS, finding a rate of 42 in 100,000 for females and 32 in 100,000 for males in New South Wales [34]. No clear-cut epidemic was observed.

In October 1985, Salit reported 50 cases from the Toronto area; 28 appeared to be linked to an infectious cause, 16 to Epstein-Barr virus (EBV) [35]. Comparable reports of CFS patients from the United States in the mid-1980s also concentrated on the Epstein-Barr question, but no true epidemic was described [36,37]. The recent epidemic in Nevada is fully described by Komaroff in Chapter 2.

CLINICAL PICTURE

This account of selected epidemics reveals several common threads. The illness is nonfatal and relapsing, affecting especially young females. A coincident known viral epidemic in the same community may or may not occur. Symptoms and signs reflect widespread involvement of the nervous system with motor, sensory, autonomic, and behavioral features. The dysfunction does not fit well into currently known patterns of nervous system involvement and deficits are not severe enough to result in objectively measurable deficits, suggesting that neurons are impaired but not killed.

In spite of many hundreds of cases and certain clear clinical patterns, the study of these epidemics does not serve to define the syndrome adequately [38]. Many questions remain. Physiologic, virologic, and biochemical data need to be gathered. Subsequent chapters will present the currently available data, and we hope the reader can reach a fuller sense of understanding.

Based on the epidemics, one can at least tease out the usual clinical features of CFS. For simplicity the symptoms may be grouped as follows.

Chronic, Lasting Fatigue

Research criteria [39] insist upon a duration of 6 months. Normal life experience exposes us to three types of fatigue: one follows unaccustomed physical exertion; another, intense sustained mental effort; the third follows inadequate sleep. The CFS patient suffers a pernicious exaggeration of all three forms. Fatigue in the syndrome is, then, both intense and polyvalent. None of the available fatigue rating instruments, often developed for fatigue in the workplace, has found widespread use and acceptance [40–44]. The requirement of 6 months' duration of fatigue allows CFS to be distinguished from postviral syndromes (for example, influenza and infectious mononucleosis). The character of the symptom may be identical, but most people with postviral syndrome feel well again within several weeks or months. The terminology used by CFS patients to describe their fatigue often suggests muscle weakness, but in fact weakness is not a feature.

Myalgia

Sometimes fatigue is accompanied by muscle tenderness, as described by Goldenberg in Chapter 5. Those patients with severe myalgia overlap with the fibromyalgia syndrome. Not all patients have muscle pain.

Psychologic Disorder

All patients with CFS experience an inexplicable decline in their ability to cope with daily life. Often this seems to correlate with perceptions of personality change, difficulty in concentrating, apparent memory disorder, and mood swings. No component of the syndrome has been as difficult to describe or delineate. Few patients have had adequate psychiatric or psychologic testing. Skeptics have advanced the view that CFS is equivalent to neurosis plus depression (if sporadic) or to mass hysteria (if epidemic). Much evidence and opinion are available to counter this skepticism, as summarized by Rogers and Chang in Chapter 3.

Authors who have seen patients with epidemic CFS comment on the following features.

1. Confusion, impairment of memory, and difficulty in concentrating are common. These symptoms, grouped together, suggest a confusional state—a disorder of cognitive function of a diffuse, nonlocalized nature. Confusional states are seen with metabolic encephalopathy, exposure to drugs or alcohol, or lesions of the brain that do not usually have a specific cortical regional distribution. In CFS the confusion is often noted to be variable and evanescent, which is compatible with a nonanatomic disorder of brain function. Patients with confusional state, owing to the associated disorder of sequential consecutive thinking, have trouble with arithmetic or with recent and intermediate memory.

2. Patients are described as labile; they may break into tears without provocation or be euphoric. Some are irritable, or described as "changed" by friends and family.

3. Depression occurs sometimes, but not often. It differs somewhat from primary typical depression in that anhedonia, anxiety, psychomotor retardation, and insomnia are uncommon. Depressive symptoms more closely resemble those seen with chronic medical or neurologic illnesses. Hypochondriasis is common: patients may bring long lists of symptoms to their clinic visits.

4. A small minority of patients have neurologic signs such as ataxia, paresis, extensor plantar response, or nystagmus. These signs are often short lived and do not in any sense "explain" the remainder of the syndrome. In the recent epidemic in Nevada, 8% of patients had such signs. In the Akureyri outbreak in Iceland, where poliomyelitis was the major concern, 28% showed weakness. Rare convulsions have occurred.

5. Formal neuropsychologic testing has not often been carried out. In patients with confusion and difficulty concentrating, it is unlikely to be particularly helpful. In the original report of the recent Nevada cases, psychologic test data were reported for 19 patients [45]. Attention, full-scale IQ, and verbal memory were affected the most (more than 60% were below norms).

DIAGNOSTIC PROBLEMS

The foregoing list of symptoms does not clearly define an entity. All observers who have worked with these patients are aware of the problems in diagnosis. Table 1–1 outlines the differential diagnoses and emphasizes that a detailed and perceptive history, basic physical examination, and minimal laboratory assessment serve to make the diagnosis. Associated complaints may broaden the differential problem,

Table 1-1. Differential considerations for CFS

Metabolic/toxic disorders
  Diabetes mellitus
  Hyperthyroidism (especially in the elderly)
  Hypothyroidism
  Hyperparathyroidism
  Addison's disease
  Hyperaldosteronism
  Hypopituitarism
  Hypercalcemia
  Alcoholism
  Chronic caffeine withdrawal state
  Drugs (see Chapter 14 for an extensive list), but especially beta blockers
    and interferon
  Anemia (tiredness may depend on the rate of development)
  Chronic electrolyte imbalance
Other general medical problems
  Chronic cardiac insufficiency
  Occult malignancy (especially lymphoma and gastrointestinal tumors)
  Connective tissue disorders
  Uremia
  Hepatic insufficiency
  Nutritional inadequacy (dieting fads, homelessness)
Infections
  Brucellosis
  Tuberculosis
  Lyme disease
  AIDS
  Mononucleosis
  Bacterial endocarditis
  Chronic pyelonephritis
  Hepatitis
  Parasitic infections
Neurologic disease
  Postconcussion syndrome
  Multiple sclerosis
  Parkinsonism
  Post-polio syndrome
  Exertion muscle pain syndrome (relieved by calcium channel blockers)
Psychiatric disease
  Depressive episode (*DSM III-R* 296.2)
  Hypochondriasis (*DSM III-R* 300.7)
  Somatization disorder (Briquet's syndrome) (*DSM III-R* 300.81)
  Generalized anxiety (*DSM III-R* 300.02)
  Malingering (*DSM III-R* V-65.20)
Physiologic causes
  Boredom
  Prolonged stress (caring for an incapacited loved one; combat)

and an algorithmic decision tree approach has been developed by Solberg [46]. The place of certain causes for chronic fatigue remains uncertain and anecdotal. Examples include poorly cleaned wall-to-wall

carpets [47], chronic overactivity of the vagal-parasympathetic system [48], chronic hypoglycemia [49], and the yeast connection [50]. Specific blood tests may simplify the problem in the near future [51]. Various authors in this monograph will present their recommendations for evaluation of patients in whom the diagnosis of CFS is being considered. Some areas of potential confusion are as follows.

Endocrine Disorder

Hyperthyroidism or hypothyroidism and hyperadrenocorticism are examples. A generation ago, many patients displaying constant fatigue, difficulty in concentrating, and myalgia would naturally have gravitated to the department of endocrinology. Advances in the field have made it possible to measure most relevant hormone levels and the patients have now become someone else's responsibility, often the neurologist's.

One need also recall the malaise, weakness, and lassitude of the person who is hypercalcemic because of parathyroid adenoma, or the muscle weakness and irritability of the patient with Cushing's syndrome.

Primary Psychiatric Disease

The relevant entities here are primary depressive disorder and one of the somatoform disorders (including conversion reaction and classical hysteria, or Briquet's syndrome). It was of great interest to us, in reviewing the data on epidemics of the past few decades, how great a source of concern the question of psychiatric disease was to the observers. Since then, psychiatric diagnostic criteria have tightened and the issues now are somewhat different. However, there is little doubt that a certain proportion of patients observed in an epidemic of CFS, and probably a larger proportion of patients with sporadic illness, are in fact psychiatric patients. They are drawn to the diagnosis of CFS because it provides them a nonpsychiatric explanation for their symptoms.

No one knows what these proportions are. Starting from the single symptom of fatigue presenting to a general physician, one study found that no more than 3 to 4% of patients will have CFS [52]. Patients referred to specialists (neurologists, psychiatrists, or rheumatologists) will have different proportions, representing the bias effect of referral patterns. For instance, Wood et al. reported that, in comparison to patients with primary muscle disease, there was more depression in a group of CFS patients and 41% could be identified as having a psychiatric disorder [53]. Imprecise diagnosis may also be at fault. CFS, myalgic encephalomyelitis (in Britain), effort syndrome, and postviral fatigue syndrome may or may not overlap or be identical.

Multiple Sclerosis

Fatigue is a prominent and sometimes early symptom of MS. As a separate symptom it is easiest to observe in mild, relapsing/remitting cases with little neurologic disability [54]. Such patients may also have relatively extensive cognitive or behavioral disorders [55]. Difficulty in separating such patients from those with CFS is obvious; we have seen errors in both directions. Some patients with a diagnosis of CFS, typically self-referred to a medical center with that diagnosis, have been found to have unequivocal evidence of demyelinating disease. Usually this consists of a magnetic resonance imaging (MRI) scan showing large, well-defined subcortical lesions, especially in the cerebellar peduncles, visible in T_2-weighted sequences. As discussed by Komaroff (Chapter 2) and Schwartz (Chapter 4), there is evidence that some patients with CFS have MRI changes. These appear to differ from those of typical MS. Nevertheless, there can be ambiguity. Measurement of visual evoked response or of spinal fluid immunoglobulin G, or cell count (both normal in CFS), can be helpful.

We have also seen patients referred with a diagnosis of MS who had fatigue, myalgia, mental change, and normal head MRI, and who were better described by the label of CFS. This is unfortunate since the treatments available are more successful for MS than for CFS.

In every epidemic of CFS, it seems obvious that some patients with early MS will be mislabeled and included as CFS. One of the two autopsies available from the Royal Free Hospital epidemic of 1955, in fact, showed changes of MS that were diagnosed during life [21].

Postviral Syndrome

In some classifications, these syndromes may arbitrarily be separated or considered part of a spectrum [56, 57]. There was confusion in the early 1980s about the role of prior Epstein-Barr virus (EBV) infection in CFS. It is now agreed that anti-EBV titers in CFS are the same as in controls or only slightly higher.

Rheumatologic Diseases

Rheumatoid arthritis, lupus erythematosus, and scleroderma are potential sources of diagnostic trouble, especially in CFS patients who do not have arthralgia or arthritis and in whom blood tests for connective tissue disease, by definition, are normal.

RELATION OF EPIDEMIC TO SPORADIC ILLNESS

The early cases of CFS were recognized because they occurred in large groups over a relatively short period. This allowed observers, particularly when the cases were institution based (Los Angeles in 1934, Royal Free Hospital in 1955), to recognize a common pattern. However, diagnosis through epidemic practically guarantees that cases falling outside the pattern will go unrecognized. This fact is especially valid for patients who have the illness in a nonepidemic pattern or when cases in an epidemic are widely scattered to many health care providers.

An estimate of 39.6 cases per 100,000 has been made for the prevalence of CFS in New South Wales [34]. How accurate is this estimate? Does it overestimate by being too inclusive and encompassing patients—presumably mostly psychiatric patients—who prefer that diagnosis to another? Or does it underestimate because many patients who truly have CFS have atypical symptoms that are not recognized? A quite different prevalence of 127 per 100,000 was calculated for New Zealand [32]. The authors of that work were well aware of these pitfalls. In the absence of answers, their estimates stand as the best available data.

RELATION OF RESEARCH CRITERIA TO PATIENTS SEEN IN PRACTICE

Three sets of research criteria, designed to guide investigators in the field, have been proposed. In the United States, the two major criteria consist of onset of disabling fatigue lasting more than 6 months and exclusion of all other potential causes [39]. Minor criteria include fever, sore throat, lymphadenopathy, muscle weakness or myalgia, headache, sleep disturbance, and neuropsychologic complaints. To make the diagnosis, the examiner should find both major criteria and 8 of 11 minor criteria (or 6 of 11 if fever, pharyngitis, or lymphadenopathy is found) (Table 1–2).

Criteria from the United Kingdom [57] and from Australia [58] differ somewhat, and in the work derived from the Oxford Conference several subcategories were developed (Table 1–3). The practicing neurologist or internist will find little value in these various research criteria. They were derived for a different purpose, which they have served. For example, inclusion of patients in studies of immune function [51] or chronic herpetic infection [59] could not be done without exclusion criteria.

However, little is gained in practice. The research guidelines do not help with the patient who has fatigue and seronegative arthralgia; or the patient with fatigue, a normal MRI, and a possible history of optic neuritis; or particularly with the patient who appears to have CFS but has a preexisting psychiatric history. According to recent reviews, more than 30% of CFS patients have such a history. Are they to be excluded from further study, as the research criteria would advise? Chapter 3 by Rogers and Chang addresses some of these issues.

Table 1-2. American research case definition of CFS

Both major criteria and either >6 symptomatic criteria plus >2 physical criteria or >8 symptomatic criteria must be present to fulfill the case definition.

Major Criteria

1. Persistent or relapsing fatigue or easy fatigability for at least 6 months that:
   a. Does not resolve with bed rest
   b. Is severe enough to reduce average daily activity by >50%
2. Other chronic clinical conditions have been satisfactorily excluded, including preexisting psychiatric diseases

Minor Criteria

Symptomatic or historical criteria: Persistent or recurring symptoms lasting >6 months:

1. Mild fever (37.5–38.6°C oral if documented by the patient) or chills
2. Sore throat
3. Lymph node pain in anterior or posterior cervical or axillary chains
4. Unexplained generalized muscle weakness
5. Muscle discomfort, myalgia
6. Prolonged (>24 hours) generalized fatigue following previously tolerable levels of exercise
7. New, generalized headaches
8. Migratory noninflammatory arthralgia
9. Neuropsychologic symptoms
   a. Photophobia
   b. Transient visual scotomas
   c. Forgetfulness
   d. Excessive irritability
   e. Confusion
   f. Difficulty thinking
   g. Inability to concentrate
   h. Depression
10. Sleep disturbance
11. Patient's description of initial onset of symptoms as acute or subacute

Physical criteria: Documented by a physician on at least two occasions, at least 1 month apart:

1. Low-grade fever (37.6–38.6°C oral or 37.8–38.8°C rectal)
2. Nonexudative pharyngitis
3. Palpable or tender anterior or posterior cervical or axillary lymph nodes (<2 cm in diameter)

Source: Modified from Holmes et al. [39].

Table 1-3. The British diagnostic guidelines for research cases

---

I. Chronic fatigue syndrome
  A. Subjective fatigue is the principal symptom of the syndrome
  B. There should be a definite onset of the syndrome (*not* life-long)
  C. Severe, disabling fatigue affects both physical and mental functioning
  D. The fatigue should have lasted for 6 months and been present 50% of the time
  E. Myalgia and disturbance of mood and sleep are common accompanying symptoms
  F. Exclusionary criteria:
    1. Established medical illnesses associated with fatigue should be excluded: a competent history and physical should be performed
    2. Psychiatric diagnoses which:
      a. Exclude CFS include schizophrenia, bipolar disease, substance abuse, eating disorder, or proven brain disease
      b. Do not necessarily exclude CFS are depressive illness, anxiety disorders, or hyperventilation syndrome

II. Postinfectious fatigue syndrome (PIFS) is considered a *subtype* of CFS that follows an infection or is associated with a current infection (although the role of an associated infection is a topic of research)

  PIFS patients must:

  A. Fulfill criteria for CFS and
  B. Have definite evidence of infection at onset (the patient's self-report per se is unlikely to be sufficiently reliable)
  C. Have the syndrome for a minimum of 6 months
  D. The infection should be corroborated by laboratory evidence

---

Source: Modified from Sharpe et al. [57].

REFERENCES

1. Hippocrates. *Complete Works*, translated by W.H.S. Jones. Cambridge, Mass.: Harvard University Press, 1968. Vol. IV, p. 359.
2. Straus, S.E. History of the chronic fatigue syndrome. *Rev. Infect. Dis.* 13: (Suppl. 1): S2, 1991.
3. Abbey, S.E., and Garfunkel, P.E. Neurasthenia and chronic fatigue syndrome. The role of culture in the making of a diagnosis. *Am. J. Psychiatry* 148:1638, 1991.
4. Beard, G.M. Neurasthenia or nervous exhaustion. *Boston Med. Surg. J.* 3:217, 1869.
5. Mitchell, S.W. *Fat and Blood: And How to Make Them (2nd ed.).* Philadelphia: Lippincott, 1882. Pp. 27–32.
6. Medoro, R., Tritchler, H.J., LeBlanc, A., et al. Fatal familial insomnia, a prior disease with a mutation to codon 178 of the prion protein gene. *N. Engl. J. Med.* 326:444, 1992.
7. Zinsser, L.T. *Rats, Lice and Men.* Boston: Little, Brown, 1934. Pp. 80–83.
8. Gilliam, A.G. Epidemiologic study of an epidemic diagnosed as poliomyelitis occurring among the personnel of the Los Angeles County General Hospital during the summer of 1934. *Public Health Bulletin*, U.S. Treasury Dept. No. 240, 1938.
9. Sigurdsson, B., Sigurjonsson, J., Sigurdsson, J.H.J., et al. A disease epidemic in Iceland simulating poliomyelitis. *Am. J. Hyg.* 52:222, 1950.

10. Sigurdsson, B., and Gundmundsson, K.R. Clinical findings six years after outbreak of Akureyri disease. *Lancet* 1:766, 1956.
11. Hyde, B., and Bergmann, S. Akureyri disease (myalgic encephalomyelitis), forty years later. *Lancet* 2:1191, 1988.
12. Pellew, R.A.A. Clinical description of a disease resembling poliomyelitis. *Med. J. Aust.* 1:944, 1954.
13. Pellew, R.A.A., and Miles, J.A.R. Further investigation on a disease resembling poliomyelitis seen in Adelaide. *Med. J. Aust.* 22:480, 1955.
14. White, D.N. and Burtch, R.B. Iceland disease: A new infection simulating acute anterior poliomyelitis. *Neurology* 4:506, 1954.
15. Acheson, E.D. Encephalomyelitis associated with poliomyelitis virus: An outbreak in a nurses' home. *Lancet* 2:1044, 1954.
16. Sumner, D.W. Further outbreak of disease resembling poliomyelitis. *Lancet* 1:764, 1956.
17. Macrae, A.D., and Galpine, J.F. An illness resembling poliomyelitis observed in nurses. *Lancet* 2:350, 1954.
18. Galpine, J.F., and Brady, C. Benign myalgic encephalomyelitis. *Lancet* 1:757, 1957.
19. Ramsay, A.M. Encephalomyelitis in northwest London. An epidemic infection simulating poliomyelitis and hysteria. *Lancet* 2:1196, 1957.
20. Ramsay, A.M., and O'Sullivan, E. Encephalomyelitis simulating poliomyelitis. *Lancet* 1:761, 1956.
21. The Medical Staff of the Royal Free Hospital. An outbreak of encephalomyelitis in the Royal Free Hospital group, London, 1955. *Br. Med. J.* 2:895, 1957.
22. Fog, T. Neuritis vegetativa epidemica. *Ugerskrift fur Laeger.* 115:1244, 1953.
23. Shelokov, A., Habel, K., Verder, E., et al. Epidemic neuromyasthenia. An outbreak of poliomyelitis-like illness in student nurses. *N. Engl. J. Med.* 257:345, 1957.
24. Hill, R.C.J. Memorandum on the outbreak amongst the nurses at Addington, Durban. *S. Afr. Med. J.* 29:344, 1955.
25. The Durban "mystery disease." *S. Afr. Med. J.* 29:997, 1955.
26. Ramsay, A.M. 'Epidemic Neuromyasthenia' 1955–1978. *Postgrad. Med. J.* 54:718, 1978.
27. Crowley, N., Nelson, M., and Stovin, S. Epidemiological aspects of an outbreak of encephalomyelitis at the Royal Free Hospital, London, in the summer of 1955. *J. Hyg.* 55:102, 1957.
28. McEvedy, C.P., and Beard A.W. Royal Free epidemic of 1955: A reconsideration. *Br. Med. J.* 1:7, 1970.
29. Poskanzer, D.C., Henderson, D.A., Kunkle, E.C., et al. Epidemic neuromyasthenia. An outbreak in Punta Gorda, Florida. *N. Engl. J. Med.* 257:356, 1957.
30. Albrecht, R.M., Oliver, V.L., and Poskanzer, D.C. Epidemic neuromyasthenia. *J.A.M.A.* 187:904, 1964.
31. Murdoch, J.C. Myalgic encephalomyelitis (ME) syndrome—An analysis of the clinical findings in 200 cases. *N.Z. Fam. Phys.* 14:51, 1987.
32. Moore, P., Snow, P., and Paul, C. An unexplained illness in West Otago. *N.Z. Med. J.* 97:351, 1984.
33. Lloyd, A.R., Wakefield, D., Boughton, C.R., and Dwyer, J.M. Immunological abnormalities in the chronic fatigue syndrome. *Med. J. Aust.* 151:122, 1989.
34. Lloyd, A.R., Hickie, I., Boughton, C.R., et al. Prevalence of chronic fatigue syndrome in an Australian population. *Med. J. Aust.* 153:522, 1990.
35. Salit, I.E. Sporadic postinfectious neuromyasthenia. *Can. Med. Assoc. J.* 133:659, 1985.

36. Straus, S.E., Tosato, G., Armstrong, G., et al. Persisting fatigue in adults with evidence of Epstein-Barr virus infection. *Ann. Intern. Med.* 102:7, 1985.
37. Holmes, G.P., Kaplan, J.E., Stewart, J.A., et al. A cluster of patients with a chronic mononucleosis-like syndrome. *J.A.M.A.* 257:2297, 1987.
38. Acheson, E.D. The clinical syndrome variously called benign myalgic encephalomyelitis, Iceland disease and epidemic neuromyasthenia. *Am. J. Med.* 4:569, 1959.
39. Holmes, G.P., Kaplan, J.R., Gantz, N.M., et al. Chronic fatigue syndrome: A working case definition. *Ann. Intern. Med.* 108:387, 1988.
40. Barofsky, I., and West, L.M. Definition and measurement of fatigue. *Rev. Infect. Dis.* 13 (Suppl. 1):S94, 1991.
41. Pearson, R.G., and Byars, G.E., Jr. The development and validation of a checklist for measuring subjective fatigue. Document No. 56115. Air University, School of Aviation Medicine, U.S. Air Force, Randolph Air Force Base, Texas, December 1956.
42. Wessely, S., and Powell, R. Fatigue syndromes: A comparison of chronic "postviral" fatigue with neuromuscular and affective disorders. *J. Neurol. Neurosurg. Psychiatry* 52:940, 1989.
43. Piper, B.F. Fatigue: Current Bases for Practice. In S.G. Funk, E.M. Tornquist, M.T. Champagne, et al. (eds.), *Key Aspects of Comfort: Management of Pain, Fatigue and Nausea.* New York: Springer, 1989. Pp. 187–198.
44. Krupp, L.B., LaRocca, N.G., Muir-Nash, J., et al. The fatigue severity scale. *Arch. Neurol.* 45:1121, 1989.
45. Daugherty, S.A., Henry, B.E., Peterson, D.L., et al. Chronic fatigue syndrome in northern Nevada. *Rev. Infect. Dis.* 13: (Suppl):S39, 1991.
46. Solberg, L.I. Lassitude: A primary care evaluation. *J.A.M.A.* 251:3272, 1984.
47. Nexo, E., Skov, P.G., and Gravesen, S. Extreme fatigue caused by badly cleaned wall-to-wall carpets. *Ecol. Dis.* 2:415, 1983.
48. Kaye, P.L. Pernicious fatigue—Identification, pathogenesis and treatment. *Physicians Drug Manual* 5:15, 1974.
49. Alexander, F., and Portis, S.A. A psychosomatic study of hypoglycemia fatigue. *Psychosom. Med.* 4:273, 1942.
50. Renfro, L., Feder, H.M., Lanet, J., et al. Yeast connection among 100 patients with chronic fatigue. *Emer. J. Med.* 86:165, 1989.
51. Landay, A.L., Jessop, C., Lennette, E.T., et al. Chronic fatigue syndrome: Clinical condition associated with immune activation. *Lancet* 338:707, 1991.
52. Manu, P., Lane, T.J., and Matthews, D.A. The frequency of the chronic syndrome in patients with symptoms of persistent fatigue. *Ann. Intern. Med.* 109:554, 1988.
53. Wood, G.C., Bentall, R.P., Gopfert, M., et al. A comparative psychiatric assessment of patients with chronic fatigue syndrome and muscle disease. *Psychosom. Med.* 21:619, 1991.
54. Krupp, L.B., Alvarez, L.A., LaRocca, N.G., et al. Clinical characteristics of fatigue in multiple sclerosis. *Neurology* 45:435, 1988.
55. Hordon, R.M. Cognitive deficits and emotional dysfunction in multiple sclerosis. *Arch. Neurol.* 47:18, 1990.
56. Behan, P.O., and Bakheit, A.M.O. Clinical spectrum of post viral fatigue syndrome. *Br. Med. J.* 47:793, 1991.
57. Sharpe, M.C., Archard, L.C., Banatvala, J.C., et al. A report—Chronic fatigue syndrome: Guidelines for research. *J.R. Soc. Med.* 84:118, 1991.
58. Lloyd, A.R., Wakefield, D., Boughton, C., et al. What is myalgic encephalitis. *Lancet* 1:1286, 1988.
59. Dale, J.K., Straus, S.E., Ablashi, D.V., et al. The Inoue-Melnick virus, human herpes virus type 6, and the chronic fatigue syndrome. *Ann. Intern. Med.* 110:92, 1989.

2

Anthony L. Komaroff

Experience with Sporadic and "Epidemic" Cases

Chronic fatigue is a common problem in general medical practice [1–4], accounting for 10 to 15 million office visits per year in the United States. It is widely believed that most cases of chronic fatigue seen in a primary care practice, or in clinics dedicated to the problem of chronic fatigue, are caused by primary psychiatric disorders. These include, particularly, depression and anxiety with somatization (psychologic or social distress expressed as bodily complaints). Indeed, many studies support that view [5–10]. On occasion, various "organic" conditions also can produce fatigue: occult malignancies or infections, inflammatory disorders of uncertain cause such as sarcoidosis, as well as anemia, thyroid disorders, multiple sclerosis, connective tissue disorders including systemic lupus erythematosus, and many other well-defined diseases. On these points most physicians would agree.

The chronic fatigue syndrome (CFS), as it has most recently been described [11–13], is not a well-defined entity. In particular, there is disagreement about whether the illness has an organic component; some observers believe that CFS is simply a condition in which certain patients with a primary psychiatric disorder describe their distress with somatic complaints. For reasons that will become apparent, I do not share that view. But it is true that, as of this writing, no etiologic agent and no characteristic pathophysiology have been identified in CFS.

Supported by the following grants from the National Institutes of Health: R01AI26788, R01AI27314, U01AI32246.

25

It does appear that CFS, as defined by the United States Centers for Disease Control (CDC) case definition (Table 2–1) [11], is an unusual cause of fatigue, accounting for fewer than 3% of all cases [14]. Moreover, it is apparent that the CDC case definition, relying as it does primarily on a group of nonspecific symptoms, may not fully meet the criteria of any case definition (i.e., the identification of a distinct group of individuals, different from people with other diseases and from people who regard themselves as healthy, and for whom reasonably accurate predictions about treatment and prognosis can be made [15]). Of course, the same is true for some well-recognized organic illnesses in which fatigue can be a prominent symptom. For example, the connective tissue disorders and multiple sclerosis can present in a less than full-blown fashion, making it impossible to diagnose these disorders definitively. Also, while the diagnosis of anemia and thyroid disease can be clear, it is not always certain whether these organic illnesses are the cause of a patient's fatigue.

SPORADIC AND EPIDEMIC FORMS

As it has been described in the literature, CFS can occur in both apparently sporadic and apparently epidemic forms. I say "apparently" because most reports of sporadic cases have not systematically assessed close contacts of the patients and because most reports of epidemic cases have not systematically evaluated the communities in which the putative epidemics occurred to determine incidental or prevalent cases.

Over the past 6 years, our group has studied a large number of patients, including what appear to be both sporadic and epidemic cases. In this chapter I summarize that experience and the tentative conclusions we are drawing from it.

Sporadic Cases

Since 1984, we have enrolled approximately 300 patients in a prospective study of CFS. The patients were referred to us by other physicians or contacted us directly after hearing about our work. Before enrolling patients in the study, we first ascertained that their symptoms and previous clinical and laboratory evaluations indicated that they might have CFS. Thus, these 300 individuals (part of a selected group) are not representative of all patients with CFS. Many of them may be more disabled by their illness than is the "typical" patient with CFS.

Each patient completed a detailed and lengthy questionnaire, had a complete physical examination (with partial neurologic examination), and underwent a battery of laboratory tests. Follow-up data (symptoms, signs, and repeat laboratory tests) were obtained for each patient. All these data are stored in a computer.

Table 2-1. Working case definition of chronic fatigue syndrome

A case of chronic fatigue syndrome must fulfill major criteria 1 and 2 and the following minor criteria: 6 or more of the 11 symptom criteria and 2 or more of the 3 physical criteria; or 8 or more of the 11 symptom criteria.

Major Criteria
1. New onset of persistent or relapsing, debilitating fatigue or easy fatigability in a person who has no previous history of similar symptoms, that does not resolve with bed rest, and that is severe enough to produce or impair average daily activity below 50% of the patient's premorbid activity level, for a period of at least 6 months.
2. Other clinical conditions that may produce similar symptoms must be excluded by thorough evaluation, based on history, physical examination, and appropriate laboratory findings. These conditions include malignancy; autoimmune disease; localized infection (such as occult abscess); chronic or subacute bacterial disease (such as endocarditis, Lyme disease, or tuberculosis), fungal disease (such as histoplasmosis, blastomycosis, or coccidioidomycosis), and parasitic disease (such as toxoplasmosis, amebiasis, giardiasis, or helminthic infestation); disease related to human immunodeficiency virus (HIV) infection; chronic psychiatric disease, either newly diagnosed by history (such as endogenous depression, hysterical personality disorder, anxiety neurosis, schizophrenia), or chronic use of major tranquilizers, lithium, or antidepressive medications; chronic inflammatory disease (such as sarcoidosis, Wegener's granulomatosis, or chronic hepatitis); neuromuscular disease (such as multiple sclerosis or myasthenia gravis); endocrine disease (such as hypothyroidism, Addison's disease, Cushing's syndrome, or diabetes mellitus); drug dependency or abuse (such as alcohol, controlled prescription drugs, or illicit drugs); side effects of a chronic medication or other toxic agent (such as a chemical solvent, pesticide, or heavy metal); or other known or defined chronic pulmonary, cardiac, gastrointestinal, hepatic, renal, or hematologic disease.

Minor Criteria
SYMPTOM CRITERIA
To fulfill a symptom criterion, a symptom must have begun at or after the time of onset of increased fatigability and must have persisted or recurred over a period of at least 6 months (individual symptoms may or may not have occurred simultaneously). Symptoms include:
1. Mild fever—oral temperature between 37.5 and 38.6°C, if measured by the patient—or chills. (*Note:* Oral temperatures >38.6°C are less compatible with CFS and should prompt studies for other causes of illness.)
2. Sore throat.
3. Painful lymph nodes in the anterior or posterior cervical or axillary distribution.
4. Unexplained generalized muscle weakness.
5. Muscle discomfort or myalgia.
6. Prolonged (24 hours or longer) generalized fatigue after levels of exercise that would have been easily tolerated in the patient's premorbid state.
7. Generalized headaches (of a type, severity, or pattern that is different from headaches the patient may have had in the premorbid state).

Table 2-1. (continued)

8. Migratory arthralgia without joint swelling or redness.
9. Neuropsychologic complaints (one or more of the following: photophobia, transient visual scotomas, forgetfulness, excessive irritability, confusion, difficulty thinking, inability to concentrate, depression).
10. Sleep disturbance (hypersomnia or insomnia).
11. Description of the main symptom complex as initially developing over a few hours to a few days (this is not a true symptom, but may be considered as equivalent to the above symptoms in meeting the requirements of the case definition).

PHYSICAL EXAMINATION CRITERIA

Physical criteria must be documented by a physician on at least two occasions, at least 1 month apart.
1. Low-grade fever—oral temperature between 37.6 and 38.6°C, or rectal temperature between 37.8 and 38.8°C. (See note under Symptom Criterion 1.)
2. Nonexudative pharyngitis.
3. Palpable or tender anterior or posterior cervical or axillary lymph nodes. (*Note:* Lymph nodes >2 cm in diameter suggest other causes. Further evaluation is warranted.)

Source: Reproduced, with permission, from G. P. Holmes, J. E. Kaplan, N. M. Gantz, et al, Chronic fatigue syndrome: A working case definition. *Ann. Intern. Med.* 108:387–389, 1988.

Among patients enrolled in the study between 1985 and October 1991, approximately 45% fully met the CDC working case definition of CFS and more than 75% met the published British [16] and Australian [17] case definitions. All had had debilitating fatigue for at least 6 months, and most had been ill for more than 3 years. Most patients had been unable to work full-time and about 20% were unable to work at all for prolonged periods.

Over 85% of the patients stated that their illness began *suddenly,* with an acute "flulike" illness characterized by fever, sore throat, cervical adenopathy, cough, abdominal symptoms, myalgias, arthralgias, and other symptoms suggesting an acute infectious process.

Symptoms

Symptoms experienced *chronically* by more than 60% of the patients with sporadic CFS included debilitating fatigue, myalgias, arthralgias, morning stiffness, sleep disorder, problems with concentration and memory, headaches, sore throat, postexertional malaise, nausea, paresthesias, irritability, and depression. From our clinical experience we believe that healthy individuals would not so frequently complain of such symptoms, but this assumption needs to be tested by polling otherwise healthy individuals and asking them the same questions in the same way. Two particularly remarkable findings are worth highlighting: chronic postexertional malaise and recurrent, often drenching night sweats (in about

40% of the patients). The night sweats were extreme, requiring changes of bedclothes and sheets. The postexertional malaise was characterized not only by symptoms that could simply represent deconditioning— pain and stiffness of the involved muscles—but also by exacerbation of "systemic" symptoms (e.g., fatigue, fevers, pharyngitis, adenopathy, and impaired cognition).

Patients with CFS stated that these symptoms and others were typ- ically *not* a chronic problem in the years before the onset of their illness, but became common after the illness began. As an example, here are the frequencies of several common chronic symptoms before and after the illness began: arthralgias, 76% vs. 6%; morning stiffness, 62% vs. 3%; distractibility, 82% vs. 4%; forgetfulness, 71% vs. 2%; dizziness, 61% vs 4%; paresthesias, 52% vs. 2%; sleep disorder, 90% vs. 7%; irritability, 68% vs. 4%; depression, 66% vs. 7%. All these symptoms are surely nonspecific, and several are thought to be concomitant symptoms of depression. However, the fact that they typically started abruptly in the context of an acute "infectious" illness suggests that the symptoms are not likely to be exclusively the result of a psychiatric disorder.

Some patients have had transient acute neurologic events: primary seizures (7%), acute, profound ataxia (6%), focal weakness (5%), tran- sient blindness (4%), and unilateral paresthesias (not in a dermatomal distribution). The clinical and laboratory findings in these relatively few patients with dramatic neurologic events are similar to those of the larger group of patients with chronic fatigue, except for the neurologic events themselves. These acute and transient neurologic events also are similar to the findings occasionally reported in outbreaks of myalgic enceph- alomyelitis.

Past Medical History
We have found a high frequency of atopic or allergic illness (in approx- imately 50%), as was first highlighted by Jones and his colleagues [18, 19] and confirmed by Straus et al. [20]. This is one of the striking findings in the past medical history of patients with CFS. In some cases, subjects developed new allergies after the onset of CFS. As discussed later in the chapter, this past atopic history may also be related to the patho- physiology of the immune response in CFS.

Physical Examination
Findings on physical examination have been relatively uncommon. We currently regard the frequency of the following physical examination findings to be unusual: approximately 35% of patients had posterior cervical adenopathy, about 10% had abnormal Romberg sign, some 20% had impaired tandem gait, and 40% could not perform serial 7s. That these findings really are abnormal needs to be confirmed by blinded examination of both patients with CFS and healthy control subjects.

Epidemic Cases

Our own experience with epidemic CFS comes from a recently published study of 259 patients who experienced the sudden onset (with a "flulike" illness) of debilitating fatigue, cognitive impairment, and many associated symptoms [21]. Their illness was consistent with the CDC case definition of CFS and is similar to past descriptions of myalgic encephalomyelitis. These patients were selected because they all sought care in the same medical practice, that is, ours was not an epidemiologic study in which a denominator population from the community was identified and studied.

Of the 259 patients, 183 lived in a particular geographic area consisting of several small towns in suburban and rural areas on and near the north shore of Lake Tahoe, in California and Nevada, and became ill within a 2-year period: they appeared to be part of an epidemic. Among these 183 patients were several "clusters" of individuals who lived or worked in close proximity: teachers and students at three different schools, co-workers at a casino, multiple family members. The other 76 were apparently sporadic instances of patients who sought care in the same practice during the same period; these patients came from urban areas of California and Nevada.

Symptoms

The patients suffered from chronic, severe debility: 29% were regularly bedridden or shut-in. More than half experienced chronic enlarged cervical lymph nodes, cough, myalgias, arthralgias, sore throat, headaches, difficulty concentrating, depression, and anxiety. As has been the case with patients from New England, fewer than 5% of the patients stated that they had experienced any of these symptoms chronically in the years before the (typically) sudden onset of their illness. The symptoms of patients in the "epidemic" group were essentially the same as those of patients in the "endemic" group.

Of the 259 patients, 22 (8%) developed evidence of an acute neurologic process: primary seizures, profound ataxia lasting several days, and paresis lasting several days. The frequency of these events was similar in the "epidemic" and "sporadic" cases.

Physical Examination

Enlarged posterior cervical nodes were found in 51% of the patients. The ataxia and paresis were confirmed during office neurologic examinations.

LABORATORY ABNORMALITIES

Because CFS currently is defined exclusively by a set of nonspecific symptoms and a few nonspecific signs, the obvious question is whether patients with CFS can be distinguished from healthy individuals by any objective laboratory data. A number of such parameters have indeed been identified in CFS, although many observations have not yet been replicated by different laboratories in different patient groups.

The next step in defining CFS as a discrete syndrome will be to see whether these laboratory abnormalities also distinguish the disorder from other well-established disease entities with which CFS can be confused: depressive disorders, somatization disorders, anxiety disorders, and mild cases of systemic lupus erythematosus or multiple sclerosis.

Standard Laboratory Evaluation

We have compared commonly obtained hematologic and chemistry tests in patients with CFS and in age- and sex-matched healthy control subjects (unpublished data). In the patients with CFS, these tests have typically been obtained on several occasions during the chronic phase of their illness, and an average value obtained for each patient.

Hematologic Testing
Several findings have been seen significantly more often in patients with CFS: lymphocytosis, atypical lymphocytosis, and (possibly) monocytosis.

Chemistry Testing
In comparison with matched healthy control subjects, our New England patients with CFS had elevated levels of alkaline phosphatase, lactic dehydrogenase, and total cholesterol. Occasional patients (perhaps 10 to 15%) had a chronic or recurrent low-grade elevation of transaminases; testing for hepatitis A, B, and C viruses was unremarkable, and there was no history of alcohol abuse or exposure to hepatotoxins.

As with the hematologic abnormalities, while each of these differences between patients and control subjects is highly significant, none of the abnormalities was seen in more than 60% of patients, and thus none serves as a useful diagnostic marker.

Immunologic Testing

A large variety of other abnormalities have been described by various investigators, but have not yet been reported by multiple laboratories studying multiple patient groups. Moreover, some conflicting results have emerged. In this regard, it is important to note that conflicting immunologic results frequently have been reported in well-defined disorders of immunity, such as HIV infection [22], multiple sclerosis, and systemic lupus erythematosus.

The abnormalities reported most consistently across multiple patient groups and in multiple immunology laboratories have been diminished function of natural killer cells [23–27], skin test anergy or impaired T-cell responses to mitogenic or antigenic stimulation [17,26,28,29], and activated T-cell subsets [26,29,30].

We and others [19,24,26,28,29,31–37] have found evidence of subtle and diffuse dysfunction: partial hypogammaglobulinemia (25–80%); partial hypergammaglobulinemia (10–30%); increased numbers of B cells; low titers of autoantibodies, particularly antinuclear antibodies (15–35%) and antibodies to single-stranded DNA; increased numbers of the subset of B cells (CD20+CD5+) that may be dedicated to the production of autoantibodies [38]; low levels of circulating immune complexes (30–50%); elevated ratios of helper/suppressor T cells (20–35%); reduced cytotoxic T-cell activity specific for Epstein-Barr virus (EBV); increased numbers of activated cytotoxic T cells; reduced in vitro synthesis of interleukin-2 and interferon by cultured lymphocytes; increased immunoglobulin E–positive cells; and elevated levels of various cytokines. Some investigators have found increased levels of circulating interferon, whereas others have not. Straus et al. demonstrated a significant increase in the activity of leukocyte 2′,5′-oligoadenylate synthetase, an enzyme induced during acute viral infections [36], although the levels were much lower than in patients with AIDS.

While the immunologic data thus far are not always consistent, and do not form a pattern that can be tied together conceptually by a unitary hypothesis, in our judgment the collective data from a growing number of well-conducted controlled studies indicate that patients with CFS are different from healthy control subjects. Indeed, the data are most consistent with the hypothesis that in CFS the immune system is chronically responding to a "perceived" antigenic challenge.

Neuropsychologic Evaluation

Formal neuropsychologic tests of cognition performed by Bastien, Albert, and their colleagues suggest that one third to one half of our patients have cognitive impairment, particularly of concentration and attention (unpublished data). It is the judgment of the neuropsychologists that the pattern of test performance suggests an "organic" deficit rather than cognitive dysfunction secondary to a mood disorder. Contrary evidence has recently been published [39].

Neuroimaging Studies

Because of the cognitive and neurologic complaints, and because of the similarity of some of these symptoms to those experienced by patients with multiple sclerosis, we have obtained magnetic resonance images (MRI) of the brain in both apparently sporadic and epidemic cases.

In the Lake Tahoe groups of apparently sporadic and epidemic cases, areas of high signal in the white matter were seen in 78% of the apparently epidemic cases, 79% of the apparently sporadic cases, and 21% of age- and sex-matched healthy control subjects, a highly significant difference ($P < 10^{-9}$)[21]. The areas of high signal typically were punctate and small, but on occasion were larger and more patchy in appearance (in none of the latter cases was there clinical or other laboratory evidence sufficient to diagnose multiple sclerosis). The subcortical white matter was affected most often, but white matter elsewhere in the central nervous system also was involved. In the few patients with a focal neurologic finding, a relationship existed between the affected anatomic area and the clinical presentation. For example, a patient with a period of ataxia lasting several days had involvement of the cerebellum, several patients with visual distortion or loss had involvement of the occipital cortex, and a patient with paresis had involvement of the contralateral internal capsule [21].

In more preliminary experience from sporadic cases in New England, we are seeing a lower frequency of MRI abnormalities: about 35 to 45% of the patients have areas of high signal in the white matter. The distribution of these areas is being compared to that in patients with multiple sclerosis and other diseases.

The meaning of these MRI abnormalities is impossible to assess without obtaining tissue. From previous experience in animals and human subjects, it is reasonable to suppose that they may represent an inflammatory process involving edema and demyelination. The areas of high signal in the subcortical white matter may also, in some instances, represent enlarged perivascular Virchow-Robin spaces. These spaces may be a normal variant, or they may represent penetration of cerebrospinal fluid into ischemic perivascular white matter or cellular infiltration into the perivascular space as part of an inflammatory process [40,41]. Based on our preliminary experience and our hypothesis that CFS is a heterogeneous process involving the interplay of different triggering agents and pathophysiologic responses, we cannot be sure whether our observations can be generalized to other patient groups who meet the criteria for CFS.

Mena (I. Mena, personal communication) and Salit (I.E. Salit, personal communication) have found perfusion abnormalities in patients studied with single-photon emission computed tomography. Our preliminary experience with about 25 patients seems to confirm this finding. It is unclear whether these abnormalities distinguish CFS from other diseases.

INFECTIOUS AGENTS AND CFS

Infectious agents have been suspected as triggering agents in CFS. Although the speculation has centered most often on viruses, nonviral infectious agents may also be able to trigger a similar postinfectious malaise [42,43].

Human Herpesvirus-6

We have evaluated the possible role of human herpesvirus-6 (HHV-6) in CFS, primarily in the Lake Tahoe patients. HHV-6 is an interesting candidate to play a pathogenetic role in some cases of CFS; it is tropic for lymphocytes, monocytes, glial cells, and neuroblastoma cells [44–48], and CFS is characterized by immunologic and neurologic symptoms. It also appears to be tropic for pulmonary and intestinal cells [48] (D.V. Ablashi, personal communication), and pulmonary and gastrointestinal symptoms are common in CFS. Our studies in association with Ablashi and Saxinger, as well as studies by others, have indicated a serologic association of this virus with both CFS and fibromyalgia [30, 49–52], although some studies have not found such an association.

Because seroepidemiologic studies suggest that infection with HHV-6 is ubiquitous and produces lifelong infection in most people beginning at a young age [53], the finding of a serologic association is not itself strong evidence of an etiologic role for HHV-6 in CFS. We therefore looked for indications that HHV-6 was actively replicating in patients with CFS. We first found such evidence in two patients, sisters who became ill at about the same time, one of whom had a dramatic lymphoproliferative syndrome [54]. Among the Lake Tahoe patients, we found a striking difference in the frequency of HHV-6 replication in patients (70%) versus healthy control subjects (20%), a highly significant difference ($P < 10^{-8}$) [21].

This finding by no means indicates that new infection with HHV-6 is a cause of CFS. New primary infection with the virus occurs early in childhood in most people [53]. Therefore for the most part, the active replication of this virus in our patients probably represents secondary reactivation rather than primary infection, and this secondary reactivation might only be an epiphenomenon. Alternatively, even if secondary, reactivated HHV-6 might play a central role in the production of CFS symptoms, as discussed later in the chapter.

Enteroviruses

For years, myalgic encephalomyelitis was thought to be produced by a less virulent strain of poliovirus. Recently several investigators have reopened the possibility that enteroviral infection may indeed be associated with some cases of CSF: circulating enteroviral antigen has been found more often in patients with CFS than in control subjects [55], and enteroviral antigen and nucleic acid are present more often in the muscle of patients with CFS than in healthy control subjects [56–58]. Of all the types of infectious agents mentioned here, the enteroviruses would seem most able to produce epidemics, adding to the plausibility that they play a role in CFS. Finally, it has now become clear that enteroviruses do not exclusively produce transient, lytic infection; they can cause a chronic, persistent form, including infection of the central nervous system [59], thus making them candidates to trigger an ongoing chronic inflammatory response such as appears to occur in CFS.

Epstein-Barr Virus

Epstein-Barr virus also has been the subject of investigation in chronic fatiguing illnesses [34–36,60]. At this time, there is little evidence to suggest that EBV is a causal agent in most cases of CFS. However, in those infrequent patients whose CFS follows in the wake of a well-documented case of acute infectious mononucleosis (about 5% of all patients, in our experience), EBV might well be playing a role in the chronic illness. Also, in those very few patients with a chronic, debilitating illness like CFS and extraordinarily abnormal antibody levels to EBV [61], the virus may also be playing a central role.

Retroviruses

We and other investigators have looked for evidence of infection with the known human retroviruses in hundreds of patients with CFS. While in a few cases, serologic evidence of infection with human T-lymphotropic virus type I or II (HTLV-I or HTLV-II) has been identified, the etiologic role of these viruses in CFS remains obscure. In a few patients who had no serologic evidence of infection with HTLV-I, HTLV-II, or human immunodeficiency virus, we have looked for reverse transcriptase in primary lymphocyte cultures to see if we could find evidence of a novel retrovirus, but without success [21].

Recently, DeFreitas and colleagues reported evidence that a novel retrovirus related to HTLV-II may be present in a large fraction of patients with CFS; this possibility has been suggested from polymerase chain reaction and in situ cytohybridization assays, although no viral cytopathic effect, no evidence of reverse transcriptase, and no electron microscopic evidence of a budding retrovirus has yet been uncovered [62]. This preliminary work, if it indeed leads to the identification of a novel retrovirus in a large fraction of patients with CFS, would be an important step forward.

One type of retrovirus, a spumaretrovirus (or "foamy virus"), has been postulated by Martin to be playing a role in CFS. As of this writing, the data have not been published or presented in detail at a scientific meeting. Research by our group has found no serologic evidence of the one known human spumavirus, human spumaretrovirus (HSRV) [63], in patients with CFS. However, if a novel spumavirus is involved in CFS, our studies might have failed to identify it.

Other Infectious Agents

A variety of nonviral infectious agents have been linked to CFS [43]. Perhaps the most persuasive data relate *Borrelia burgdorferi* to CFS. Patients with well-documented Lyme disease who have been diagnosed relatively late in the course of the illness but treated with adequate doses of antibiotics can develop a syndrome that essentially meets the criteria for CFS [64]. Interestingly, it appears that these patients have low levels of circulating immune complexes and that borrelial antigens are found within the complexes (P. Coyle, personal communication). This finding suggests that a persistent borrelial infection or a reservoir of persistent borrelial antigen may be eliciting an ongoing immunologic response characterized clinically by CFS, a hypothesis that we consider later in this chapter.

CFS AND PSYCHOLOGIC ILLNESS

The typical patient who seeks medical care for chronic fatigue must be distinguished from the relatively unusual patient with CFS. As stated at the outset, most patients seeking medical care for chronic fatigue are probably suffering from depression or anxiety (and the related condition called somatization), and do not have CFS [14,65].

The identification of antecedent or subsequent psychiatric disorders in patients who may have an underlying organic illness can be difficult. The affective disorders, not being generally measurable by an objective laboratory test, are formally defined by subjective findings: symptoms expressed by the patient and the appearance of the patient to the skilled observer. Moreover, many of the symptoms taken as characteristic of depression, anxiety, and somatization—fatigue, cognitive impairment, sleep disturbance, nausea—also are seen with a variety of organic illnesses. Therefore, patients with CFS or with well-established organic illnesses may meet the criteria for major depression without always having a depressive state.

The evidence presented earlier of objective immunologic and virologic findings that distinguish patients with CFS from healthy control subjects suggests that CFS is probably not simply a primary psychiatric disorder. However, that suggestion must be confirmed by doing similar immunologic and virologic studies on patients with primary psychiatric disorders, particularly major depression, to make sure that the findings seen in CFS patients are not just previously unrecognized biologic concomitants of depression. (Of course, if patients with major depression were found to have evidence of immunologic dysregulation and active viral replication, it could profoundly change our concepts of what psychiatric disorders are.) One piece of evidence that CFS and major depression are not the same thing is work of Demitrack and colleagues showing that abnormalities of the hypothalamic-pituitary-adrenal axis in CFS patients are entirely different from those seen in patients with major affective disorder [66].

Even if preexisting psychiatric disorders are unlikely to explain CFS fully, they can play a role in the syndrome. Every study of the question indicates that the majority of patients with CFS *become* depressed and anxious within 1 to 2 months following the (usually sudden) onset of their disorder [67–71]. For many patients, the depression and anxiety are the most debilitating parts of their illness, and such patients should be encouraged to obtain treatment for the depression and anxiety. This can be a difficult task. Some patients reject what they regard as a stigmatizing label, and many patients (and physicians) seem to divide diseases of the mind and diseases of the body into two mutually exclusive categories: For some people, it is hard to understand that an illness may have both "organic" and psychologic components.

The more difficult question is whether patients who develop CFS have had evidence of a psychiatric disorder in the years *before* their disease began or had an active psychiatric disorder *at the onset* of the CFS. We and others have used retrospective interrogation with formal instruments such as the Diagnostic Interview Schedule (DIS) to evaluate the presence of psychiatric disorders in the years before the CFS appeared [67–71]. None of these studies has carefully evaluated whether there was an active psychiatric disorder at the time of the onset. By and large, the studies find a somewhat higher past history of psychiatric disorders in patients with CFS than in the general population: The average across all studies is around 30% (range, 20–50%) of CFS patients versus 5 to 10% in the population at large [67–72]. There are at least two caveats in interpreting these reports. First, the studies vary greatly with regard to the reported relative frequencies of depression, anxiety, and somatization. Second, the published studies were largely organized and conducted before a formal case definition of CFS was developed; thus, the patients may not all meet CFS criteria and the studies may not be comparable with one another.

If a background of psychiatric disease, particularly depression, is present more often in patients with CFS, what might that mean? It could indicate that the syndrome is just depression expressed with predominantly somatic symptoms; however, the fact that most patients with CFS do not appear to have a preexisting psychiatric condition is evidence against this hypothesis. Or it could indicate that CFS is triggered by an organic illness, such as an infection, that is followed and then supplanted by the reemergence of an underlying depression; this is sometimes spoken of as the "hit-and-run" hypothesis, in which the triggering infectious agent has long since left the scene but for some reason a persisting state of depression or anxiety is left in its wake. Or it could indicate that the biologic underpinnings of depression somehow render a person vulnerable to the "organic" abnormalities (e.g., immunologic and virologic findings) seen in CFS.

We are more inclined to favor the last hypothesis, although it is not mutually exclusive with the other two. While affective disorders are surely influenced in part by life events, they also surely are biologically determined disorders of neurochemistry—disorders that can affect immune function and that, in turn, can be perturbed by the immune system. According to this model, "mind" and "body" are not separate and discrete, but inevitably linked: biologic forces that increase the likelihood of affective disorders also may increase vulnerability to disorders of immunity. In patients with CFS who have a current or past affective disorder and who also have evidence of immune dysfunction and active viral infection, it may never be possible to determine whether the affective disorder, the immune dysfunction, or the viral infection came first. Rather, the practical question is what form of management will be most effective: psychotherapy, pharmacotherapy of the affective disorder, "immune modulating" pharmacotherapy, antimicrobial therapy, or some combination. There are no good studies of these issues at present.

A MODEL FOR THE PATHOGENESIS OF CFS

Our pervasive ignorance about the pathogenesis of CFS makes possible the elaboration of many models, but provides strong support for none of them. Our current view of this illness is reflected in Figure 2-1. We think the disease is influenced by both physical and psychologic factors. And, as with any illness, the degree of disability seen in CFS must be due, in part, to physical and psychologic factors.

In our current view, CFS is primarily an immunologic disturbance that allows reactivation of latent and ineradicable infectious agents, particularly viruses. While this may be only an epiphenomenon, we believe it is more likely that, once secondarily reactivated, the viruses contribute to the morbidity of CFS—directly, by damaging certain tissues (e.g., the pharyngeal mucosa), and indirectly, by eliciting an ongoing immunologic response. In particular, the elaboration of various cytokines (e.g., interferon-α, tumor necrosis factor, interleukin-1, and interleukin-2) as part of this ongoing immunologic war may produce many of the symptoms of CFS: the fatigue, myalgias, fevers, sleep disorder, adenopathy, and even the disorders of mood and cognition. This possibility is suggested by the finding of increased levels of various cytokines in CFS and related conditions [31–33], and the experience with infusing cytokines made by recombinant DNA techniques for various therapeutic purposes [73–79].

What triggers the immune dysfunction in the first place? It is likely that many factors could do so: atopic disorders, exogenous lymphotropic

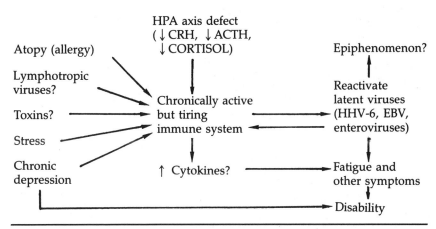

Fig. 2-1. Chronic fatigue syndrome is currently thought to be a heterogeneous illness involving complex interactions between external factors that stress the immune system and the subsequent interplay of immunologic, virologic, neurologic, and psychologic factors. These are discussed at more length in the text. (From *Post-viral Fatigue Syndrome: A Review of American Research and Practice*, by A. L. Komaroff. Copyright © 1991 by John Wiley & Sons, Ltd. Reprinted by permission of John Wiley & Sons, Ltd.)

infectious agents, environmental toxins, stress, and, as argued earlier, the biology of an underlying affective disorder. Recent research also suggests that a defect in the hypothalamic-pituitary-adrenal (HPA) axis may lead to a state of mild tertiary hypoadrenalism, which could, in turn, encourage a state of chronic immunologic activation [80]. The syndrome probably has a multifactorial origin, like most illnesses. While the discovery of a single explanation, such as a novel infectious agent or a specific inherited immunologic defect, might facilitate the search for solutions to this illness, we are dubious that such a simple answer will emerge. In any event, it is encouraging that a growing amount of research is being conducted in laboratories around the world, seeking answers for the patients with this often devastating disorder.

REFERENCES

1. Allan, F.N. The differential diagnosis of weakness and fatigue. *N. Engl. J. Med.* 231:414, 1944.
2. Morrison, J.D. Fatigue as a presenting complaint in family practice. *J. Fam. Pract.* 10:795, 1980.
3. Katerndahl, D.A. Fatigue of uncertain etiology. *Fam. Med. Rev.* 1:26, 1983.
4. Nelson, E., Kirk, J., McHugo, G, et al. Chief complaint fatigue: A longitudinal study from the patient's perspective. *Fam. Pract. Res. J.* 6:175, 1987.

5. Stoeckle, J.D., Zola, I.K., and Davidson, G.E. The quantity and significance of psychological distress in medical patients. *J. Chron. Dis.* 17:959, 1964.
6. Reifler, B.V., Okimoto, J.T., Heidrich, F.E., and Inui, T.S. Recognition of depression in a university-based family medicine residency program. *J. Fam. Pract.* 9:623, 1979.
7. Hoeper, E.W., Nycz, G.R., Cleary, P.D., et al. Estimated prevalence of RDC mental disorder in primary medical care. *Int. J. Ment. Health* 8:6, 1979.
8. Nielsen, A.C.I., and Williams, T.A. Depression in ambulatory medical patients. *Arch. Gen. Psychiatry* 37:999, 1980.
9. Kessler, L.G., Cleary, P.D., and Burke, J.D. Psychiatric disorders in primary care. *Arch. Gen. Psychiatry* 42:583, 1985.
10. Barsky, A.J.I. Hidden reasons some patients visit doctors. *Ann. Intern. Med.* 94:492, 1981.
11. Holmes, G.P., Kaplan, J.E., Gantz, N.M., et al. Chronic fatigue syndrome: A working case definition. *Ann. Intern. Med.* 108:387, 1988.
12. Straus, S.E. The chronic mononucleosis syndrome. *J. Infect. Dis.* 157:405, 1988.
13. Komaroff, A.L. The "chronic mononucleosis" syndromes. *Hosp. Pract.* 22:71, 1987.
14. Manu, P., Lane, T.J., and Matthews, D.A. The frequency of the chronic fatigue syndrome in patients with symptoms of persistent fatigue. *Ann. Intern. Med.* 109:554, 1988.
15. Komaroff, A.L., and Geiger, A. Does the CDC working case definition of chronic fatigue syndrome (CFS) identify a distinct group? *Clin. Res.* 37:778A, 1989.
16. Sharpe, M.C., Archard, L.C., Banatvala, J.E., et al. A report—Chronic fatigue syndrome: Guidelines in research. *J. R. Soc. Med.* 84:118, 1991.
17. Lloyd, A.R., Wakefield, D., Boughton, C.R., and Dwyer, J.M. Immunological abnormalities in the chronic fatigue syndrome. *Med. J. Aust.* 151:122, 1989.
18. Olson, G.B., Kanaan, M.N., Gersuk, G.M., et al. Correlation between allergy and persistent Epstein-Barr virus infections in chronic active Epstein-Barr virus–infected patients. *J. Allergy Clin. Immunol.* 78:308, 1986.
19. Olson, G.B., Kanaan, M.N., Kelley, L.M., and Jones, J.F. Specific allergen-induced Epstein-Barr nuclear antigen–positive B cells from patients with chronic-active Epstein-Barr virus infections. *J. Allergy Clin. Immunol.* 78:315, 1986.
20. Straus, S.E., Dale, J.K., Wright, R. and Metcalfe, D.D. Allergy and the chronic fatigue syndrome. *J. Allergy Clin. Immunol.* 81:791, 1988.
21. Buchwald, D., Cheney, P.R., Peterson, D.L., et al. A chronic illness characterized by fatigue, neurologic and immunologic disorders, and active human herpesvirus-6 infection. *Ann. Intern. Med.* 116:103, 1992.
22. deMartini, R.M., and Parker, J.W. Immunologic alterations in human immunodeficiency virus infection: A review. *J. Clin. Lab. Anal.* 3:56, 1989.
23. Aoki, T., Usuda, Y., Miyakoshi, H., et al. Low natural killer syndrome: Clinical and immunologic features. *Nat. Immun. Cell Growth Regul.* 6:116, 1987.
24. Caligiuri, M., Murray, C., Buchwald, D., et al. Phenotypic and functional deficiency of natural killer cells in patients with chronic fatigue syndrome. *J. Immunol.* 139:3306, 1987.
25. Kibler, R., Lucas, D.O., Hicks, M.J., et al. Immune function in chronic active Epstein-Barr virus infection. *J. Clin. Immunol.* 5:46, 1985.
26. Klimas, N.G., Salvato, F.R., Morgan, R., and Fletcher, M. Immunologic abnormalities in chronic fatigue syndrome. *J. Clin. Microbiol.* 28:1403, 1990.

27. Whiteside, T.L., and Herberman, R.B. The role of natural killer cells in human disease. *Clin. Immunol. Immunopathol.* 53:1, 1989.
28. Murdoch, J.C. Cell-mediated immunity in patients with myalgic encephalomyelitis syndrome. *N.Z. Med. J.* 101:511, 1988.
29. Gupta, S., and Vayuvegula, B. A comprehensive immunological study in chronic fatigue syndrome. *Scand. J. Immunol.* 33:319, 1991.
30. Landay, A.L., Jessop, C., Lennette, E.T., and Levy, J.A. Chronic fatigue syndrome: Clinical condition associated with immune activation. *Lancet* 338:707, 1991.
31. Wallace, D.J., Margolin, K., Waller P. Fibromyalgia and interleukin-2 therapy for malignancy. *Ann. Inter. Med.* 108:909, 1988.
32. Peter, J.B., and Wallace, D.J. Abnormalities of immune regulation in the primary fibromyalgia syndrome. *Arthritis Rheum.* 31:24, 1988.
33. Cheney, P.R., Dorman, S.E., and Bell, D.S. Interleukin-2 and the chronic fatigue syndrome. *Ann. Intern. Med.* 110:321, 1989.
34. DuBois, R.E., Seeley, J.K., Brus, I., et al. Chronic mononucleosis syndrome. *South. Med. J.* 77:1376, 1984.
35. Jones, J.F., Ray, C.G., Minnich, L.L., et al. Evidence for active Epstein-Barr virus infection in patients with persistent unexplained illnesses: Elevated anti-early antigen antibodies. *Ann. Intern. Med.* 102:1, 1985.
36. Straus, S.E., Tosato, G., Armstrong, G., et al. Persisting illness and fatigue in adults with evidence of Epstein-Barr virus infection. *Ann. Intern. Med.* 102:7, 1985.
37. Tosato, G., Straus, S., Henle, W., et al. Characteristic T cell dysfunction in patients with chronic active Epstein-Barr virus infection (chronic infectious mononucleosis). *J. Immunol.* 134:3082, 1985.
38. Casali, P., Burastero, S.E., Nakamura, M., et al. Human lymphocytes making rheumatoid factor and antibody to ssDNA belong to Leu1 + B-cell subset. *Science* 236:77, 1987.
39. Altay, H.T., Abbey, S.E., Toner, B.R., et al. The neuropsychological dimensions of postinfectious neuromyasthenia (chronic fatigue syndrome): A preliminary report. *Int. J. Psychiatry Med.* 20:141, 1990.
40. Jungreis, C.A., Kanal, E., Hirsch, W.L., et al. Normal perivascular spaces mimicking lacunar infarction: MR imaging. *Radiology* 169:101, 1988.
41. Heier, L.A., Bauer, C.J., Schwartz, L., et al. Large Virchow-Robin spaces: MR-clinical correlation. *A.J.N.R.* 10:929, 1989.
42. Rosene, K.A., Copass, M.K., Kastner, L.S., et al. Persistent neuropsychological sequelae of toxic shock syndrome. *Ann. Intern. Med.* 96:865, 1982.
43. Salit, I.E. Sporadic postinfectious neuromyasthenia. *Can. Med. Assoc. J.* 133:659, 1985.
44. Salahuddin, S.Z., Ablashi, D.V., Markham, P.D., et al. Isolation of a new virus, HBLV, in patients with lymphoproliferative disorders. *Science* 234:596, 1986.
45. Josephs, S.F., Salahuddin, S.Z., Ablashi, D.V., et al. Genomic analysis of the human B-lymphotropic virus (HBLV). *Science* 234:601, 1986.
46. Ablashi, D.V., Salahuddin, S.Z., Josephs, S.F., et al. HBLV (or HHV-6) in human cell lines. *Nature* 329:207, 1987.
47. Komaroff, A.L. Human herpesvirus 6 and human disease. *Am. J. Clin. Pathol.* 93:836, 1990.
48. Levy, J.A., Ferro, F., Lennette, E.T., et al. Characterization of a new strain of HHV-6 (HHV-6SF) recovered from the saliva of an HIV-infected individual. *Virology* 178:113, 1990.
49. Buchwald, D., Saxinger, C., Goldenberg, D.L., et al. Primary fibromyalgia (fibrositis) and human herpesvirus-6: A serologic association. *Clin. Res.* 36:332A, 1988.

50. Komaroff, A.L., Saxinger, C., Buchwald, D., et al. A chronic "post-viral" fatigue syndrome with neurologic features: Serologic association with human herpesvirus-6. *Clin. Res.* 36:743A, 1988.
51. Krueger, G.R.F., Ablashi, D.V., Josephs, S.F., et al. Clinical indications and diagnostic techniques of human herpesvirus-6 (HHV-6) infection. *In Vivo* 5:287, 1991.
52. Ablashi, D.V., Josephs, S.F., Buchbinder, A., et al. Human B-lymphotropic virus (human herpesvirus-6). *J. Virol. Methods* 21:29, 1988.
53. Saxinger, C., Polesky, H., Eby, N., et al. Antibody reactivity with HBLV (HHV-6) in U.S. populations. *J. Virol. Methods* 21:199, 1988.
54. Buchwald, D., Freedman, A.S., Ablashi, D.V., et al. A chronic "postinfectious" fatigue syndrome associated with benign lymphoproliferation, B-cell proliferation, and active replication of human herpesvirus-6. *J. Clin. Immunol.* 10:335, 1990.
55. Yousef, G.E., Bell, E.J., Mann, G.F., et al. Chronic enterovirus infection in patients with postviral fatigue syndrome. *Lancet* 1:146, 1988.
56. Archard, L.C., Bowles, N.E., Behan, P.O., et al. Postviral fatigue syndrome: Persistence of enterovirus RNA in muscle and elevated creatine kinase. *J. R. Soc. Med.* 81:326, 1988.
57. Cunningham, L., Bowles, N.E., Lane, R.J.M., et al. Persistence of enteroviral RNA in chronic fatigue syndrome is associated with the abnormal production of equal amounts of positive and negative strands of enteroviral RNA. *J. Gen. Virol.* 71:1399, 1990.
58. Gow, J.W., Behan, W.M.H., Clements, G.B., et al. Enteroviral RNA sequences detected by polymerase chain reaction in muscle of patients with postviral fatigue syndrome. *Br. Med. J.* 302:692, 1991.
59. Sharief, M.K., Hentges, R., and Ciardi, M. Intrathecal immune response in patients with the post-polio syndrome. *N. Engl. J. Med.* 325:749, 1991.
60. Tobi, M., Morga, A., Ravid, Z., et al. Prolonged atypical illness associated with serologic evidence of persistent Epstein-Barr virus infection. *Lancet* 1:61, 1982.
61. Schooley, R.T., Carey, R.W., Miller, G., et al. Chronic Epstein-Barr virus infection associated with fever and interstitial pneumonitis: Clinical and serologic features and response to antiviral chemotherapy. *Ann. Intern. Med.* 104:636, 1986.
62. DeFreitas, E., Hilliard, B., Cheney, P.R., et al. Retroviral sequences related to human T-lymphotropic virus type II in patients with chronic fatigue immune dysfunction syndrome. *Proc. Natl. Acad. Sci. USA* 88:2922, 1991.
63. Flugel, R. Spumaviruses: A group of complex retroviruses. *J. Acquir. Immune Defic. Syndr.* 4:739, 1991.
64. Coyle, P.K., and Krupp, L.B. *B. burgdorferi* infection in the chronic fatigue syndrome. *Ann. Neurol.* 28:243, 1990.
65. Kroenke, K., Wood, D.R., Mangelsdorff, A.D., et al. Chronic fatigue in primary care: Prevalence, patient characteristics, and outcome. *J.A.M.A.* 260:929, 1988.
66. Demitrack, M.A., Dale, J.K., Gold, P.W., et al. Neuroendocrine abnormalities in patients with chronic fatigue syndrome. *Clin. Res.* 37:532A, 1989.
67. Taerk, G.S., Toner, B.B., Salit, I.E., et al. Depression in patients with neuromyasthenia (benign myalgic encephalomyelitis). *Int. J. Psychiatry Med.* 17:49, 1987.
68. Kruesi, M.J.P., Dale, J., and Straus, S.E. Psychiatric diagnoses in patients who have chronic fatigue syndrome. *J. Clin. Psychiatry* 50:53, 1989.
69. Wessely, S., and Powell, R. Fatigue syndromes: A comparison of chronic "postviral" fatigue with neuromuscular and affective disorders. *J. Neurol. Neuorsurg. Psychiatry* 52:940, 1989.

70. Hickie, I., Lloyd, A., Wakefield, D., and Parker, G. The psychiatric status of patients with the chronic fatigue syndrome. *Br. J. Psychiatry* 156:534, 1990.
71. Gold, D., Bowden, R., Sixbey, J., et al. Chronic fatigue: A prospective clinical and virologic study. *J.A.M.A.* 264:48, 1990.
72. Robins, L.N., Helzer, J.E., Weissman, M.M., et al. Lifetime prevalence of specific psychiatric disorders in three sites. *Arch. Gen. Psychiatry* 41:949, 1984.
73. Muss, H.B., Costanzi, J.J., Leavitt, R., et al. Recombinant alpha interferon in renal cell carcinoma: A randomized trial of two routes of administration. *J. Clin. Oncol.* 5:286, 1987.
74. Quesada, J.R., Talpaz, M., Rios, A., et al. Clinical toxicity of interferons in cancer patients. *J. Clin. Oncol.* 4:234, 1986.
75. Erstoff, M.S., and Kirkwood, J.M. Changes in the bone marrow of cancer patients treated with recombinant interferon alpha 2. *Am. J. Med.* 76:593, 1984.
76. Rosenberg, S.A., Lotze, M.T., Muul, L.M., et al. A progress report on the treatment of 157 patients with advanced cancer using lymphokine activated killer cells and interleukin 2 or high dose interleukin 2 alone. *N. Engl. J. Med.* 316:889, 1987.
77. Belldegrun, A., Webb, D.E., Austin, H.A.I., et al. Effects of interleukin 2 on renal function in patients receiving immunotherapy for advanced cancer. *Ann. Intern. Med.* 106:817, 1987.
78. Denicoff, K.D., Rubinow, D.R., Papa, M.X., et al. The neuropsychiatric effects of treatment with interleukin 2 and lymphokine activated killer cells. *Ann. Intern. Med.* 107:293, 1987.
79. Ettinghausen, S.E., Puri, R.K., and Rosenberg, S.A. Increased vascular permeability in organs mediated by the systemic administration of lymphokine activated killer cells and recombinant interleukin 2 in mice. *J. Natl. Cancer Inst.* 80:178, 1988.
80. Demitrack, M.A., Dale, J.K., Straus, S.E., et al. Evidence for impaired activation of the hypothalamic-pituitary-adrenal axis in patients with chronic fatigue syndrome. *J. Clin. Endocrinol. Metab.* 73:1223, 1991.

3

Malcolm P. Rogers
Grace Chang

Psychiatric Aspects

Chronic fatigue syndrome (CFS) is an enigmatic disease that has defied pathophysiologic clarification and confounded doctor and patient alike. In particular, psychiatric disease such as depression or somatization disorder may produce symptoms similar to those of CFS. In order to provide an operational definition of CFS as the basis for clinical and epidemiologic research, the Centers for Disease Control (CDC) has devised major criteria for CFS that require exclusion of both newly diagnosed and preexisting chronic psychiatric disease [1]. Whether such a restricted definition will ultimately help unravel the puzzle of this disorder remains to be seen. In any event, it has not stopped continued speculation about the relationship of psychiatric disorder to CFS, both in the research and the clinical sphere.

CASE VIGNETTE: "JANICE"

One way to highlight some of the issues and dilemmas facing clinicians in treating patients with CFS is to start with a clinical example:

> At the time of her referral to a psychiatrist, "Janice" was a 33-year-old divorced mother of one with a diagnosis of CFS. She was referred by her rheumatologist at her own request for help in coping with her chronic illness.
> She had been sickly as a child, with a pattern of frequent viral infections, sore throats diagnosed as "strep," swollen glands, and low-grade fevers. She

was even given penicillin prophylactically, but the recurrent pharyngitis continued.

In high school she was bothered by migratory arthralgias and myalgias that sometimes interfered with her participation in sports and other activities. At 15, an apparent diagnosis of "mono" was made, and she was out of school and bedridden for 3 months. She recalls that whenever she tried to exert herself, she would feel very bad the next day. During late high school and early college years, all of these symptoms persisted but were less severe: sore throat, swollen glands, low-grade fevers (99.6–101°F), arthralgias, and myalgias. In fact, she became very athletic, pushing herself to the extreme of running in marathons, although she recalled that she would feel terrible for some time after such vigorous activity.

Around the age of 29 or 30, the arthralgias became more severe and headaches began. She experienced a number of tick bites around this time. She also had an episode of hives and respiratory distress for which she was treated in an emergency ward. Thereafter, she had persistent fatigue and cognitive difficulties, and worsening of all the previous symptoms. The cognitive difficulties included poor word recall and diminished memory, more pronounced when she was more fatigued. She also began to have spells characterized by loss of consciousness for several minutes, typically preceded by a rush of dysesthesias on the skin of her legs, moving upward toward the trunk, arms, and head, followed by slurred speech, mood lability with weeping, mental "fogginess," visual distortions, dizziness, and inability to walk without support. These spells were not associated with any jerking movements, tongue biting, or incontinence.

All of these symptoms, especially the fatigue, made it increasingly difficult for her to continue her job as a manager in a company, and within a few months of the referral she had left work on a disability leave.

In terms of objective findings, her physical examination has been normal on almost all occasions except for the presence of one skin nodule on her forearm. A biopsy revealed "panniculitis with perivascular lymphocytic infiltrate of uncertain type and cause." She has a moderate anemia (hematocrit 32–35) with normal iron, total iron-binding capacity, ferritin, vitamin B_{12}, folate, and lead levels. Otherwise, her chemistry and serologic studies have been essentially normal. Computed tomography of the abdomen and pelvis, chest roentgenogram, and echocardiogram were all negative.

Neurologic testing revealed possible mild bilateral neuropathy on nerve conduction studies of the lower extremities (absent H wave bilaterally). Of two electroencephalograms, one revealed rare theta activity in the left temporal region and the other, bitemporal atypical theta activity, both of questionable significance.

"Janice" was the second oldest of four children. She described both parents as being critical and cold to the point of emotional neglect; on occasion, they were verbally and even physically abusive. Her father was described as a stoic engineer who rarely expressed any affection or support. Her mother had been more critical and erratic as a parent. She had experienced two "nervous breakdowns" during which bizarre and perhaps even psychotic behavior emerged, but she never obtained formal psychiatric treatment.

"Janice" had been a good athlete and student with artistic inclinations.

While in college, she married and had a daughter. The baby was ill at birth with symptoms of projectile vomiting, epilepsy, and recurrent infections, and underwent several workups for a possible autoimmune disorder. No definite diagnosis was ever made, and her daughter gradually recovered. However, the strain of this illness contributed to the dissolution of the patient's marriage. The only previous psychiatric treatment she had received was marriage counseling and, later, help for her daughter around her adjustment to the divorce.

At the time of the referral, "Janice" was functioning as a single parent and trying to maintain her job despite diminishing stamina. Most of her energy went into "surviving a demanding schedule" with little support from her parents.

At the initial psychiatric evaluation, she did not present with a major depressive episode but rather with depressive symptoms more typical of a situational adjustment reaction. She did not appear to be deriving secondary gain from her illness. She was taking 50 mg of amitriptyline, which afforded some improvement in her sleep pattern. The ongoing conflicts with her parents might have led her into useful psychotherapeutic work regardless of the CFS. However, she discontinued treatment for about one and a half years before returning.

In the interim she had taken a disability leave from her job, remarried, and given birth to a second child. Over this period her husband had become less communicative and less supportive to her. The pattern of her symptoms was essentially unchanged except perhaps for the addition of intermittent diarrhea, loss of appetite and other gastrointestinal symptoms, and worsening of her prior cognitive symptoms. These now included episodic slurring of speech, difficulty with dates, trouble remembering names and phone numbers, and diminished concentration that caused her to "re-read something several times before it registered."

Neuropsychologic testing showed evidence of psychomotor slowing in some areas such as the Continuance Performance Test. The psychologist thought this change was most likely secondary to depression. Since he also observed that she was not experiencing any depressive affects per se, he believed this would have to be an "occult or atypical depression."

However, there were also some focal neuropsychologic deficits including decay of verbal information and dichotic digit testing characteristic of left temporal lobe dysfunction. He also thought that the verbal/performance discrepancy (99/109) indicated impairment of the dominant hemisphere. Since she had no history of learning disability and reported that her verbal SAT score had been higher than her math, the neuropsychologist considered these changes significant.

This brief clinical vignette raises many questions about the interaction between psychiatric illness and CFS. In the remainder of the chapter, we will attempt to answer these questions based on the available scientific literature.

Did this patient have a prior psychiatric condition? How many patients with CFS have a premorbid psychiatric disorder? How do we measure it? Did this patient have a longstanding organic illness, either CFS or some other disorder, or was the early somatic symptomatology simply reflective of a longstanding somatoform disorder? Could there have been an occult or masked depression? Is that a valid diagnostic entity? Was her daughter genetically predisposed to a similar pattern of illness, or was this somatoform disorder by proxy? [2].

From a psychodynamic perspective, what is the significance of her feeling of being neglected and emotionally abused by her parents? Does this have a bearing on possible primary or secondary gain from her illness? Has illness served a purpose in her life, albeit unconscious, to elicit care and concern to compensate for its early absence? Or is her illness a symbolic representation or repetition of her sense of suffering alone amidst the failure of others to relieve it? If one looks deeply enough for such possible hypotheses or psychodynamic issues, are they not always present to some degree?

What about the impact of the illness on her emotional and mental state? If it can sometimes produce cognitive and other neurologic changes, as seems to be the case here, what direct effects might it have on mood and mentation? How do we differentiate changes which may be part and parcel of the underlying disease from those which occur as a reaction to the disease? What would be the impact of having a disease whose validity remains doubtful to so many in and out of the medical profession? What is the psychologic impact on the patient when a physician questions the validity of his or her symptoms, or of the disease itself? What does that do to the doctor-patient relationship? On the other hand, does labeling the syndrome a disease reinforce the sick role or prolong disability?

Consider the referral to a psychiatrist. When should a referral be made? In this case, the patient requested it. If she had not, at what point and in what manner should the primary physician raise the issue or explicitly recommend it? To whom should the patient be referred and for what type of treatment?

PREVALENCE OF PSYCHIATRIC ILLNESS IN CFS

Research strategies investigating the relationship of CFS and psychiatric disorder have relied on the concept of choosing a defined group of patients. Possible groups to be considered would be:

1. Patients who adhere to a research definition of CFS, presumably a small subset of the whole; for instance, patients with prior psychiatric history, or prior episodes of CFS, or prior family history, or poorly defined inflammation such as arthritis. In using such a group of strictly defined CFS patients, one assumes that the small subset adequately represents the whole.

2. Patients with fatigue from any source, who can be assessed to obtain the prevalence of CFS. In so doing, one can investigate the various groups of patients with fatigue, some with CFS, others with thyroid disease, hepatic disease, multiple sclerosis, inflammatory arthritis, and so forth. CFS patients could be compared with the other groups along various dimensions such as prevalence of psychiatric disorders, level of function, severity of fatigue, and other signs and symptoms.

3. Patients with known and defined psychiatric illness, for instance those with major depression or dysthymia, who can be compared with strictly defined CFS patients. Are their signs, symptoms, and laboratory findings similar? Is the cognitive deficit the same or different? What about family history?

4. Patients who are part of a CFS epidemic. Epidemics of CFS furnish some validity to the idea that the condition does exist. What psychiatric problems have been experienced by patients in the epidemic forms of CFS? What are the prognostic implications?

Cases Defined by CDC Criteria

In a study of 135 consecutive patients with 6 or more months of debilitating fatigue who presented to the Chronic Fatigue Clinic of the University of Connecticut Health Center, Manu and colleagues applied the CDC consensus definition of CFS [3]. The patients were also evaluated by a complete history, physical examination, a comprehensive battery of blood tests, and the Diagnostic Interview Schedule (DIS), a highly structured interview that generates psychiatric diagnoses according to the current edition of the *Diagnostic and Statistical Manual of the American Psychiatric Association (DSM III-R)*. It should be noted that the majority of patients (123, or 91%) were self-referred and that there was no control group of medical outpatients without chronic fatigue.

These internal medicine researchers found that six of the 135 subjects (4%) satisfied diagnostic criteria, whereas 91 (67%) of the patients had clinically active psychiatric disorders and four (3%) had medical problems that accounted for their fatigue. The authors concluded that CFS is infrequent among patients with symptoms of persistent fatigue.

In a report released simultaneously, the same researchers described the psychiatric morbidity of 100 subjects complaining of chronic fatigue with a mean duration of 13 years, using the procedures already described [4]. Of the 66 patients with one or more psychiatric diagnoses considered to be a major cause of their fatigue, 47 had a mood disorder, 15 had a somatization disorder, and nine had an anxiety disorder.

Finally, in an expanded study of 200 adults with the chief complaint of chronic fatigue, the same investigators at the same clinic, using the same comprehensive medical and psychiatric assessment, found that 13% of the patients satisfied the diagnostic criteria for panic disorder, a frequency 10-fold that found in the general population [5]. Moreover,

21 of the 26 patients had panic disorder that either preceded or was coincidental with the onset of chronic fatigue.

In each of these studies, Manu and his colleagues made observations about a population of patients with complaints of chronic fatigue who sought help at the chronic fatigue clinic of a university hospital. They were not studying a group which met the consensus definition of CFS; in fact, only 4% did.

In a recent study by other investigators, the prevalence of psychiatric disorders among 98 patients with chronic fatigue was similarly high in 19 patients who met CDC criteria for CFS and 79 who did not [6]. Both groups were compared to a control group of 31 patients with rheumatoid arthritis along a battery of structured psychiatric interviews and questionnaires. Patients with chronic fatigue had a significantly higher lifetime prevalence of major depression and somatization disorder than the patients with arthritis. In over half the patients, the psychiatric illness preceded the onset of chronic fatigue.

Cases Assessed by a Psychiatric Diagnosis

Alternative research strategies have been used to investigate the psychiatric status of patients with CFS. For example, Kruesi and co-investigators assessed the lifetime prevalence of psychiatric disorders using the DIS in a sample of 28 patients who met CDC case definition criteria for CFS and who had unusual Epstein-Barr virus (EBV) profiles [7]. All 28 subjects were seropositive for EBV and were eligible for a placebo-controlled acyclovir treatment trial at the National Institutes of Health. Twenty-one of the 28 patients (75%) satisfied diagnostic criteria for psychiatric illness. In only two patients (10%) did the onset of chronic fatigue occur 1 year or more before any psychiatric problem, whereas CFS followed psychiatric illness in 10 of the 21 cases (48%). The lifetime prevalence of major depression was 46% in this sample. The authors reported 10% rates for somatization disorder and antisocial personality disorder among women subjects. For all three disorders, the rates reported are higher than those in the general population. While these findings are provocative, the small sample size and potential sample bias owing to the drug study requirements may limit their applicability to CFS patients without EBV seropositivity.

Krupp and her co-investigators also studied a sample of CFS patients and found a higher prevalence of psychiatric disorders than would be expected in a general community sample [8]. Using a self-report questionnaire, the Million Multiphasic Clinical Inventory (MMCI-II), to generate *DSM III-R* diagnoses, Krupp and co-investigators found that 65 to 75% of their subjects had either an Axis I or Axis II (personality disorder) diagnosis. No information was provided about how long these disorders may have been present and, specifically, whether they preceded or followed the onset of CFS. However, anxiety disorder was the common

Axis I diagnosis and compulsive personality disorder the most common for Axis II. Although the incidence of psychiatric disturbances was high, they also emphasized that 25 to 35% of CFS patients did not have a diagnosable psychiatric disorder, suggesting that, at least in a sizable subgroup of CFS patients, psychologic factors do not play a role.

Some researchers have argued that because the CDC criteria specifically exclude patients with psychiatric disorders, accurate quantification of psychologic symptoms in CFS patients is precluded [9]. Accordingly, Hickie and his co-investigators compared 48 CFS subjects (not requiring exclusion because of a history of psychiatric illness) with 48 psychiatric patients diagnosed as having nonendogenous depression on a number of psychometric measures. While the interviewing psychiatrist was not blind to the CFS status of the study participants, the premorbid prevalence of major depression (12.5%) and lifetime psychiatric illness of CFS subjects (24%) did not exceed general community prevalence estimates. In comparison to depressed controls, the CFS patients did not have a high premorbid rate of psychiatric disorder, were significantly less neurotic, and showed different psychiatric symptoms. In addition, the CFS patients demonstrated high scores on disease conviction: an attitude of determined certainty about the presence of disease and resistance to reassurance. The authors concluded that psychologic disturbance is a consequence of CFS. They did find a high incidence of coexisting major depression during the course of illness in CFS patients: 22 of the 48 patients, or 46%.

Differences in attributions and self-esteem in depressed and CFS patients have been reported by other investigators. For example, Powell and co-workers found that CFS patients (subjects who had 6 or more months of fatigue without demonstrated organic cause) tended to attribute their symptoms to external causes while depressed controls had inward attribution [10]. Their CSF patients had little self-blame or lowered self-esteem and appeared to satisfy diagnostic criteria for depression on the basis of mood change, sleep and appetite disturbance, somatic symptoms, and anhedonia. These differences raise serious questions about the validity of the diagnosis of major depression in CFS patients.

In contrast to patients with neuromuscular disorders such as myasthenia gravis and myopathy, CFS patients have greater "mental fatigue"—fatigue precipitated by mental effort—and associated cognitive difficulties [11]. A control group of depressed patients was similar in their reports of mental fatigue, but less likely than the CFS patients to attribute it to physical causes.

COGNITIVE IMPAIRMENT

Cognitive dysfunction has been another prominent symptom in patients with CFS and, unlike a history of psychiatric disorders, has not been a criterion for exclusion. In fact, listed as minor CDC criteria for CFS are the following "neuropsychologic complaints": photophobia, transient visual scotomas, forgetfulness, irritability, confusion, difficulty thinking, inability to concentrate, and depression [1]. Some investigators have doubted that such cognitive complaints represent organic brain disturbance. Altay and his group reported on the neuropsychologic dimensions of postinfectious neuromyasthenia (PIN) [12]. All 21 subjects who sought treatment for this illness met CDC criteria for CFS. Subjects were administered standard neuropsychologic tests to assess their complaints of impaired attention, concentration, and abstraction skills. In fact, the researchers found that their PIN/CFS patients scored significantly better than age-matched norms on tests of concentration, attention, and abstraction, perhaps underscoring the discrepancy between subjective complaints of cognitive impairment and the objective test results. On the other hand, the highly educated subjects in this study had a mean 16.5 years of education. A comparison of their performance before and after PIN/CFS and with control groups matched for education might allow more definitive conclusions.

Other investigators have been more impressed with the cognitive dysfunction associated with CFS, and demonstrated the impairment—and sometimes improvement—by neuropsychologic testing [13]. In several series of patients, around 50% present symptoms of difficulty concentrating, dyslogia, and memory impairment [14,15]. Some have found the most prominent area of dysfunction to be retrieval of information and set switching and attention. Others have emphasized the difference between these cognitive changes and those seen in major depression, and underscored the need for more rigorous attention to methodology in their measurement [16].

THE ISSUE OF DEFINING PSYCHIATRIC DISORDER IN THE MEDICALLY ILL

Many clinicians and researchers have long pointed out the difficulties of accurately diagnosing psychiatric disorders in the presence of medical illness. Affective and somatoform disorders pose particular difficulties in this regard. Both operational definitions include many somatic symptoms. In both cases, inclusion of these somatic symptoms in support of the psychiatric diagnosis depends on the conclusion that they are not attributable to an underlying medical disorder. In the case of major depression, for example, if fatigue, insomnia, anorexia, and loss of concentration can be accounted for by a medical illness, they cannot be counted as evidence for the diagnosis of depression. This overlapping of symptoms has led others to propose different criteria for the diagnosis of depression in medically ill patients—criteria which emphasize cognitive and mood changes as opposed to somatic symptoms [17]. Abbey and her co-workers found a cluster of self-report symptoms from the Beck Depression Inventory (BDI), which are best able to identify major depression in medically ill patients: self-hate, indecisiveness, loss of appetite, and suicidal thoughts [18]. Obviously, the decision whether to count or discount somatic symptoms in reference to *DSM III-R* definitions of depression, even in research-oriented, structured diagnostic interviews, is a matter of interpretation by the interviewer. In the study by Powell et al., the absence of diminished self-esteem and increased self-blame in CFS patients who met *DSM III-R* criteria for major depression raised questions about the meaningfulness of the diagnosis, especially since their somatic symptoms could be attributed to their medical disorder.

Perhaps the approach taken by Krupp and her colleagues represents the most useful way of proceeding [19]. Rather than using *DSM III* definitions of depression, they utilized a self-report scale, the Center for Epidemiologic Studies Depression Scale (CES-D), which emphasizes the affective component of depressive symptoms. They compared CFS patients and other groups of patients with medical disorders in which fatigue is a major symptom—multiple sclerosis, systemic lupus erythematosus, Lyme disease—as well as healthy volunteers. All subjects underwent a thorough neurologic examination in addition to the CES-D Scale and the Fatigue Severity Scale (FSS). All disease groups had significantly higher CES-D ratings of depression than the normal controls, and CFS subjects had significantly higher scores than each of the other groups. The authors point out that depression may be more common than previously thought in medical disorders in which fatigue is a major symptom. FSS scores were significantly higher in patients with disease than in the healthy control group and, again, significantly higher in the CFS group. Across all groups, measures of depression and fatigue were significantly correlated. The authors stress the importance of including medical illnesses that involve prominent fatigue as appropriate control groups for CFS; otherwise, depression levels in CFS will be misleadingly higher than in other medical illnesses.

A similar conundrum applies to somatoform disorders. If any of the various symptoms in somatization disorder or somatoform pain disorder are commensurate with and attributable to an identified medical illness, then by definition they are not included as evidence of a somatoform disorder. Such clinical judgments are notoriously difficult for trained interviewers using structured diagnostic interviews, and hardly easier for the most skilled clinician. In our case vignette, for example, whether "Janice's" somatic symptoms in childhood and adolescence were early symptoms of CFS or were, instead, part of a pattern of somatization disorder is a toss-up. It is interesting that she lacked the affective features shown best to predict a major depression episode [18].

THE ISSUE OF PSYCHOLOGIC CAUSALITY

CFS as a Somatoform Disorder

What conclusions can be reached concerning the causal role of psychologic factors or psychopathology in CFS? There is really very little hard data pertaining to this question but no shortage of speculation and opinion, some of it highly politicized. For example, in a recent controversial article, two Toronto researchers, Susan Abbey and Paul Garfinkel, draw a parallel between the nineteenth century's neurasthenia and the current diagnosis of CFS [20]. They argue that CFS is a psychiatric problem resulting from chronic stress that is made culturally acceptable by being viewed as a medical disorder. They suggest that stress encountered in the workplace from rapidly changing technologies and gender conflicts arising from the rapidly changing role of women in our society are important psychosocial causes in the development of CFS, much as they were in the similar syndrome of neurasthenia appearing at the end of the nineteenth century. The 1989 study by Kruesi et al. [7] of 28 subjects who were all seropositive for EBV found that 48% had a history of psychiatric disorder *preceding* the onset of CFS. In contrast, in only 10% of the cases did CFS begin 1 year or more before onset of the psychiatric disorder. The study by Katon et al. [6] also found a high prevalence of psychiatric disorders that *preceded* the onset of chronic fatigue in over half the cases, although only a minority of their patients met criteria for CFS. On the other hand, in one of the few additional attempts specifically designed to answer the question, Hickie and co-workers [9] reached exactly the opposite conclusion. Comparing 48 CFS patients to normal population controls and to a group of patients with nonendogenous depression, they concluded that the prevalence of psychiatric disorder *prior* to the onset of CFS was no higher in the CFS group than in the population controls. In contrast, the control group with nonendogenous depression had more psychiatric disorder and was more neurotic than the CFS group. This study includes a more appropriate sample of CFS patients (not excluding a history of psychiatric illness), but its methodology is somewhat flawed by the lack of blinded evaluation. The generality of Kruesi's study is limited by its use of a CFS subgroup with positive EBV serology. All of the studies rely on *DSM III* definitions of psychiatric disorders, although it is probable that Hickie interpreted the same criteria differently.

Thus, the issue of whether or not there are predisposing psychologic characteristics or an increase in premorbid psychiatric disorders cannot be answered definitively from these studies. It is doubtful that further progress will be made in delineating the role of depression unless it is defined by more appropriate criteria for those with prominent physical symptoms—namely, with an emphasis on affective and cognitive features of depression [18,19]. Furthermore, the exclusion of psychiatric history in the CDC definition of CFS is likely to obfuscate the matter further unless exceptions to the definition are made, as Hickie and colleagues [9] have done.

There are other hypotheses, as yet untested by rigorous study. One is that the premorbid personality profile of CFS patients is one of a "high-achieving," "hard-driving," and athletic nature [21]. Whether this profile predisposes toward the development of CFS or simply to a higher likelihood of distress and treatment seeking among those who become ill is unclear.

Based on long-term follow-up of a 1955 epidemic of myalgic encephalitis [22], one investigator has speculated that CFS may be a form of mass hysteria or conversion disorder [23]. The epidemic affected nurses and doctors at the Royal Free Hospital in London, producing a syndrome similar to CFS. In a 13-year case control–designed follow-up study, the affected nurses showed more neuroticism, experienced more illness prior to the onset of the epidemic, and had more subsequent psychiatric contact than the control group. Of course, whether or not the initial epidemic was psychogenic can only be a matter of guesswork, and one could attribute the increased neuroticism and psychiatric treatment to the secondary psychologic sequelae of the epidemic illness.

CFS as an Affective Disorder

If there has been speculation that CFS is really just a recent culturally determined version of a somatoform disorder [20,24], there has been even more speculation that it represents an affective disorder in disguise. The notion of "masked depression," presenting with more somatic than affective or cognitive symptoms of depression, is a longstanding clinical concept—indeed, in our case vignette the idea of "occult" depression was raised. As a concept, it predates the *DSM III* and *DSM III-R* era of descriptive and operational definitions of psychiatric disorders, and perhaps would find a place in the current nomenclature under the category of atypical depression.

However, additional evidence suggests that CFS is different from, and not a manifestation of, an affective disorder. For one thing, the characteristically shortened REM latency—time from sleep onset to the first period of rapid eye movement (REM) sleep—associated with major depression has not been observed. Instead, Moldofsky has found prolonged REM latency and an increase in alpha-delta sleep, or what he has referred to as "unrefreshing sleep," a pattern similar to that observed in fibromyalgia [25]. Krupp and Mendelson [26] reported an increase in sleep apnea and periodic leg movements in patients with CFS. Indeed, in polysomnographic sleep studies, Krupp found abnormalities in 7 of 10 CFS patients that she believed might be making a significant contribution to their symptoms.

Another marker for major depression has been dysregulation of the hypothalamic-pituitary-adrenal axis, most frequently measured with the dexamethasone suppression test. Preliminary studies on CFS patients have not revealed abnormal levels of corticotropin-releasing hormone, further suggesting that major depression is not masquerading as CFS [27].

The Link Between CFS and Psychiatric Disease

Overall, one would have to conclude from these studies that there is little hard evidence to support the notion that CFS is essentially psychogenic in origin, as a manifestation of either a somatoform or an affective disorder. On the contrary, some evidence directly refutes this hypothesis, and, as other chapters in this volume attest, there is growing evidence for immunologic and neurologic disturbance in the syndrome.

On the other hand, notwithstanding the definitional issues, there may be an increased prevalence of psychiatric disorders among CFS patients, as several studies have suggested. There does appear to be an increased level of psychopathologic disturbance among patients with fatigue symptoms who come to medical centers and specialized chronic fatigue clinics. Perhaps this should not be surprising. We already know, for example, that there is an increased prevalence of a wide range of psychiatric disorders in primary care and general practice settings. That it might be even higher among a group of patients whose illness has eluded medical diagnosis and effective treatment is not surprising. An additional possibility is that CFS itself produces psychiatric illness, not just as a secondary reaction, but by directly involving the central nervous system. The neurocognitive symptoms certainly highlight this possibility.

It may well turn out instead that there is an increase in the prevalence of some psychiatric disorders prior to the development of CFS, whether an affective disorder, an anxiety disorder such as panic disorder, a somatoform disorder, or even particular personality disorders or traits. If so, the question will be whether the disorder predisposes patients to CFS or simply reflects a more general, perhaps even genetic vulnerability. In our case vignette, even if "Janice" does not have a preceding somatoform disorder, she clearly comes from a dysfunctional family. Perhaps such subclinical but developmental risk factors may be more significant than preceding *DSM III-R* diagnoses. Not infrequently, individuals deprived of love and affection, or even physically abused, at an early age unconsciously seek the care and attention derived from the sick role, or repeat some aspect of their childhood experience through their illness. "Janice's" life, quite apart from her CFS, has been unusually difficult and painful. On a cautionary note, it should be remembered that if one looks hard enough for areas of conflict that might underlie somatic symptoms, one can usually find them.

There may well be distinctive differences in the pattern and course of CFS between various subgroups, such as those who have comorbid psychiatric disorders or preceding subclinical psychologic difficulties and those who do not. Moreover, the secondary development of psychiatric symptoms, either affective or cognitive, may have important implications for prognosis as well.

THE PSYCHOLOGIC IMPACT OF CFS

Virtually all observers, whether patients or doctors, have commented on the profound psychologic impact of having this disorder. Not only do the symptoms often disrupt the entire pattern of a patient's life—from work to relationships to recreation to finances—but they challenge his or her basic integrity and self-concept.

Issue of Lack of Validation

Consider a recent editorial written by Dr. Thomas English, a physician, himself struggling with CFS [28]:

> Skepticism permeates our profession. It is ingrained during medical training and reinforced by professional experience . . . Healthy skepticism is the "in" attitude for intelligent, discriminating physicians.
> But healthy for whom?
> Four years ago I was diagnosed as having chronic fatigue syndrome (CFS). The experience has given me a new perspective of my profession, one that is not always flattering. In one early report the average CFS patient had previously consulted 16 different physicians. Most were told that they were in perfect health, that they were depressed, or that they were under too much stress. Many were sent to psychiatrists. The situation is better today, but not by much . . .
> Is CFS a real disease? I believe it is, but I cannot settle that here. I would only plant this seed in the mind of skeptics: *What if you are wrong?* What are the consequences for your patients?
> Imagine for a moment that you are the Subjective patient, not the Objective physician. You catch a "cold" and thereafter the quality of your life is indelibly altered. You can't think clearly . . . sometimes it's all you can do to read the newspaper or follow the plot of a television program. Jet lag without end. You inch along the fog-shrouded precipice of patient care, where once you walked with confidence. Myalgias wander about your body with no apparent pattern. Symptoms come and go, wax and wane. What is true today may be partially true tomorrow or totally false next week. You know that sounds flaky, but, dammit, it's happening to you.
> You are exhausted, yet you can sleep only two or three hours a night. You were a jogger who ran three miles regularly; now a walk around the block depletes your stamina. Strenuous exercise precipitates relapses that last weeks. *There is nothing in your experience in medical school, residency, or practice with its*

grueling hours and sleep deprivation that even approaches the fatigue you feel with this illness. "Fatigue" is the most pathetically inadequate term.

You too might wonder about some of your symptoms had you not talked to other patients with similar experiences . . . or talked with physicians who have seen hundreds of similar cases. . . .

I have talked with scores of fellow patients who went to our profession for help, but who came away humiliated, angry, and afraid. Their bodies told them they were physically ill, but the psychospeculation of their physicians was only frightening and infuriating—not reassuring. It told them their doctors had little understanding of the real problem. Many patients had depleted themselves financially, dragging in vain through expensive series of tests and consultants as their lives crumbled around them. They had lost careers, homes, families, in addition to the loss of stamina and cognitive skills. *There is nothing that you hold dear that this illness cannot take from you. Nothing . . .* (Reprinted, with permission, from *J.A.M.A.* 265:964, 1991. Copyright 1991, American Medical Association.)

In one way or another, almost all patients deal not only with the losses resulting from the illness, but from a perceived lack of credibility with the medical profession. They have formed support groups, organized on a national level as the Chronic Fatigue and Immune Dysfunction Syndrome Association (CFIDS) with local chapters throughout the nation. Newsletters from the central organization and district chapters reflect the distress over lack of validation that many patients feel. Most of the publications from the CFIDS community contain a mixture of updated medical information, reports of meetings, patient letters, and personal stories. They are laced with humor and cartoons, often biting, which provide patients an opportunity to respond to the powerlessness and anger they may have felt when interacting with the medical profession. For example, one newsletter contains a holiday greeting in the form of a cartoon. Santa Claus, stripped to the waist and looking bedraggled, is sitting in a doctor's office on the examining table, as the doctor examines the chart and announces "It seems you have CFIDS, Mr. Claus. Since I don't believe you or it exists, I suggest you see another doctor." Another cartoon has a patient crawling to the doctor's office, then sitting slumped in a chair as the cheerful doctor says, "You couldn't be that tired . . . you managed to get here!" [29].

The very name of the organization, Chronic Fatigue and Immune Deficiency Syndrome Association, is an attempt to emphasize the validity of the illness. For most patients and many doctors working in this area, the word *fatigue* does not seem to capture the severity of the symptom or the syndrome, as Dr. English points out in his editorial [28]. Sufferers of the disorder have also had to fight disparaging labels such as "Yuppie flu."

Unpredictability

The uncertainty and unpredictability of the disease are also a major part of what makes it so disruptive. This is not a new observation. For years, patients with chronic autoimmune disorders such as multiple sclerosis, rheumatoid arthritis, and systemic lupus erythematosus have spoken and written about the difficulty of planning work and social activities because they could not be certain they would feel well enough on any particular day to honor their commitments. Reasonably conscientious people would rather promise nothing than promise something they cannot deliver. The fluctuation and uncertainty typifying CFS is an underappreciated aspect of what makes it so disruptive and disabling. Once again, Dr. English speaks to this aspect of the disease when he says, "Symptoms come and go, wax and wane. What is true today, may be partially true tomorrow, or totally false next week" [28].

Disability

There is no doubt that CFS is often disabling. In fact, one study has documented that 45% of the subjects were periodically bedridden [30]. Yet, despite their often disabling symptoms, many patients have a difficult time convincing insurance companies or the Social Security Administration that they should receive disability benefits. There is nothing visible or tangible about most of their limiting symptoms, whether fatigue or cognitive impairment, and relatively few objective findings.

Within the CFIDS association, individuals have tried to help fellow patients and even their physicians in preparing the required reports and documentation of their illness. Detailed reports, thoroughly documenting the symptoms and basis for the diagnosis of CFS are helpful, as well as detailed descriptions of the limitation in activities. Even so, most patients with CFS are turned down on their first or second application for Social Security Disability; if they win their case, it is usually on appeal before an administrative law judge.

Supporting their patients' claim for disability is difficult for most physicians. Not only is it time consuming, but the process often seems in direct conflict with central tasks of the physician—namely, promoting health and trying to improve function. At the very least, physicians are often ambivalent about verifying or predicting prolonged disability for a patient (it has to last for at least 1 year to qualify for Social Security disability). Physicians may worry that they are reinforcing the sick role and disability, making eventual recovery a longer, more arduous process. They may even feel that patients are using them, consulting with them in the first place in order to document their inability to function, not necessarily in pursuit of recovery. On the other hand, patients legitimately unable to work need financial support. They need their physician to be a strong ally and advocate on their behalf. Physicians need to remind themselves that their most basic role is the relief of suffering.

MANAGEMENT

Dr. Gantz's chapter contains an overall discussion of the management of CFS (Chapter 14). Our focus here is primarily on psychologic management.

When and How to Refer to a Mental Health Specialist

Most patients are eager to discuss the impact of the disease on their lives and psychologic well-being. Many patients would gladly accept the opportunity to have such a discussion in more depth with a psychiatrist or psychologist, provided that they felt their medical illness was not being invalidated in the process. CFS patients are extremely sensitive to the implication that the disease is "all in their head," (i.e., not real but imagined). The best way to make a successful referral is to emphasize that the patient's physical complaints are being taken seriously and will continue to be thoroughly investigated and monitored. At the same time, a patient's mood and level of stress often can affect his or her body and capacity to cope with such an illness. Therefore, the referral to a psychiatrist is part of the overall care of the patient and attempts to utilize every approach that might provide some relief from suffering. It is an attempt to be thorough and to treat the "whole person," a concept most patients can readily accept.

The process is certainly easier when the patient initiates the request for a referral. If this does not happen, however, who should be referred? Probably not everyone, but certainly patients who have significant symptoms of depression, or anxiety, or cognitive impairment; also, patients who appear to have other major stresses in their lives, an inadequate support network, or a premorbid psychiatric disorder. Even if a past history of psychiatric disorder raises the possibility of a psychogenic basis for the patient's symptoms, the referral should still emphasize the potential benefit of improved coping. The alliance in the referral process should be made around the psychologic impact of the disease. In most cases, the possibility of psychologic factors in the onset of CFS would need to be explored indirectly with emphasis on alleviating whatever psychologic distress might be aggravating the symptoms.

To whom should the patient be referred? In most cases to a psychiatrist, who would have the broadest view of diagnosis and treatment and would be prepared to initiate or recommend psychopharmacologic intervention, if warranted. If individual psychotherapy is needed, other psychotherapists such as psychologists, social workers, or nurse practitioners might be appropriate. For questions of cognitive impairment, patients will need to be referred to psychologists skilled in neuropsychologic testing.

Psychologic Testing

Detailed neuropsychologic testing, in the hands of a skilled psychologist, may be one of the best ways of clarifying and documenting the extent of cognitive impairment. It can be important for several reasons. First, it may be one of the most objective indicators of a disease process in CFS. For such an elusive disease, any objective documentation is important. Second, it is important for most patients to differentiate between self and disease. Patients literally ask, "Is that me or is that my disease?" Preservation of a clear sense of self provides a necessary foundation for coping with any disorder. Third, it may be important to document for purposes of disability determination, since cognitive impairment may become the most disabling aspect of the disease for some patients. Fourth, learning in more detail which cognitive functions are impaired may have important explanatory benefits for patients and allow for developing compensatory strategies as well as ways of avoiding situations in which a particular cognitive difficulty will put them at the greatest disadvantage [31]. Many patients learn to keep more written notes or directions and to avoid being in crowded, noisy groups where acquiring new information is most difficult.

Other Testing: MRI, SPECT, BEAM

There are usually several different specialists involved in the care of a patient with CFS, any of whom might order further neuropsychiatric studies. As mentioned elsewhere in the volume, there is emerging evidence of changes evident on brain magnetic resonance imaging (MRI) or on single-photon emission computed tomography (SPECT) scanning. Mena's SPECT scan studies of CFS patients showed a reduction in blood flow to the temporal lobes and, to a lesser extent, to the frontal and parietal lobes as well [32]. MRIs have revealed punctate areas of high signal in the subcortical white matter of the brain [33]. Brain electrical activity mapping (BEAM) may also represent a promising area for further study. Goldstein's preliminary work suggests frequent abnormalities in the right posterior temporal region of many CFS patients [34]. For the same reasons that it is important to document objective neurocognitive changes in this elusive disease, changes in brain structure and function must be recorded as well. While it might be frightening to some patients, and rarely leads to specific interventions, it is more often reassuring for patients to know that their symptoms are derived from identifiable brain changes. The down side is in finding questionable changes of uncertain significance.

If the patient has seen an internist, a neurologist, and a psychiatrist, it is obviously important that these physicians communicate among themselves so as best to coordinate care in general, and specifically to coordinate any neurologic and neuropsychiatric tests.

The Role of Psychotherapy

Although there are few studies documenting the benefits of psychotherapy, either individual or group, for patients with CFS, much anecdotal evidence supports its usefulness. For other chronic medical conditions such as rheumatoid arthritis [35] or breast cancer [36], such evidence does exist, largely for structured group therapy. Not only has such intervention led to greater quality of life and reduction in pain, but in some cases it has been associated with reductions in objective indicators of disease severity and even with prolongation of life [36].

Most of these interventions have been structured and psychoeducational in nature, have contained a mixture of support with enhancement of self-efficacy or a sense of control, and have presented specific techniques for controlling pain or coping with other aspects of the illness experience. The more directive psychotherapeutic approaches are often aimed at cognitive restructuring or specific behavioral approaches such as relaxation, self-hypnosis, and exercise. Both cognitive and behavioral approaches have been successfully applied to patients with CFS [37,38]. The cognitive restructuring has been focused on getting patients to reinterpret the meaning of physical symptoms—in particular, to stop assuming that such symptoms always mean tissue damage. It also seeks to modify the behavior that often follows such misinterpretation, namely, the avoidance of any physical activity associated with an increase in these symptoms.

Most of these same approaches could be used in individual psychotherapy as well, but some patients may derive specific benefits from a group experience. Meeting with other CFS patients is likely to reduce feelings of isolation and provide a sense of validation. Self-help groups do not offer the range of approaches available in a structured program led by a well-trained mental health specialist. However, they are inexpensive and widely available through chapters of the CFIDS Association; patients should be made aware of this organization for the general network of support and information it provides. Individual psychotherapy is indicated for treatment of significant depression or anxiety problems, or in dealing with specific issues that have unique effects on individual patients.

Other Nonspecific Approaches

Adapting to CFS requires major changes in a patient's life. Patients need to pace themselves and to learn to readjust their expectations about what they can accomplish in a given time period. They need to discipline themselves not to push to their upper limits, and to get an adequate amount of rest, so that they can be sure to accomplish their priorities. Many patients will push too hard when they are having a better day, only to suffer the consequences for several days afterward. Often they need to redefine their priorities. Excessive stress should be eliminated. Many patients find that lying down to rest for a period each day helps to preserve their energy. Keeping a daily log may identify patterns adversely affecting fatigue, or vice versa, and may also help to evaluate the effects of various interventions.

Exercise is important in preventing the kind of fatigue that results form deconditioning. The exercise does not have to be strenuous. Even if it involves only a few minutes of walking daily to begin with, it can gradually be lengthened to 5 minutes and then increased in very small increments. Bicycling and swimming may be added as stamina permits.

The overall strategy of assuming a greater sense of control over the rhythm of everyday life is an important step in reducing the uncertainty that can be so erosive.

The Role of Psychoactive Medications

Antidepressants

Patients with symptoms of major depression will benefit from an adequate course of an antidepressant, particularly one with few sedative effects such as nortriptyline (Pamelor) [39] bupropion (Wellbutrin) [40] or fluoxetine (Prozac). Bupropion appears to have special efficacy in the subtype of major depression characterized by extreme fatigue and hypersomnia [41]. However, antidepressants rarely lead to a dramatic recovery from all somatic symptoms, especially fatigue, in the average CFS patient. The failure of most patients to fully recover their energy after a course of antidepressants is further evidence that CFS is not simply another form of major depression. Used judiciously, however, antidepressants often have a beneficial effect. They may have some other target symptoms as well, generally in lower doses. The tricyclics have an analgesic effect independent of their antidepressant effect. Amitriptyline has been used most frequently in this regard, not just for CFS but also for fibromyalgia, a closely related disorder. Its sedative effect also seems to help in maintaining sleep. Others have recommended low-dose doxepin (Sinequan), the most sedating of the tricyclics. Some have recommended its use in combination with a benzodiazepine to help in sleep onset—either clonazepam (Klonopin) 0.5 mg or alprazolam (Xanax) 0.25 mg. For all patients, assuming they do not have a total fear or aversion to the use of medications, a trial-and-error period to find the right medication or drug combination is important.

Stimulants

Although there are no reported studies of stimulants in the treatment of CFS, some investigators have suggested the use of pemoline or amantadine, both of which have been given to counteract the fatigue associated with multiple sclerosis [42,43].

Anxiolytics

Given the preliminary evidence that the prevalence of panic and other anxiety disorders is increased in patients with CFS, the high-potency benzodiazepines clonazepam (Klonopin), alprazolam (Xanax), and lorazepam (Ativan) may be of particular benefit. For generalized or nonspecific anxiety problems, however, it is not advisable to have CFS patients taking benzodiazepines on a long-term basis. The lethargy and sedation associated with their use should be avoided.

Benzodiazepines may be of benefit in sleep-onset insomnia, particularly for short-term use. If insomnia is a major problem for a patient with CFS and does not appear to be primarily a function of a major depressive episode, an all-night sleep study using polysomnography should be considered to rule out apnea, nocturnal myoclonus, restless legs, or narcolepsy.

Another possible role for benzodiazepine might be as an adjunct in the management of a chronic pain syndrome, especially when tricyclics have failed or increased muscle tension appears to be a contributing mechanism.

CASE VIGNETTE REVISITED

Let us reconsider the earlier case of "Janice" in light of the known literature. Did she have a premorbid psychiatric disorder? The answer is still ambiguous. If we conclude that her earlier, varied somatic symptoms could not be attributed to a medical disorder, then there are enough symptoms to meet *DSM III-R* criteria for somatization disorder; if we conclude otherwise, the diagnosis of somatization disorder melts away. Se we are left with the same fundamental dilemma.

Yet, in terms of the alliance that seems essential for any positive therapeutic effect, the practical answer is clear: Since this patient has an unshakable conviction that there is a physical basis for her symptoms, to suggest or even imply a psychologic cause would be to undermine our rapport with her. And if we were wrong in that approach, we would have added to her suffering, as many other patients have so poignantly explained. What if we were wrong in the opposite direction? Would we be reinforcing her illness or her sick role? Our guess is that seeming to doubt the validity of her symptoms would only encourage her to convince us otherwise, which would probably intensify the symptoms, or maybe just disrupt the relationship. Of course, from a psychiatrist's point of view, symptoms are no less real even if their origin is psychogenic, but many patients would not appreciate the subtlety of this distinction.

In any event, it is certainly possible to accept and empathize with the patient's explanatory model of the illness while silently considering other hypotheses. What is the impact of her family's neglectful and sometimes emotionally abusive treatment? What was the quality of her early relationships, and how might that be contributing to her CFS? These are important dynamic considerations that can be explored without directly challenging her own perception of her current illness. In fact, the process of therapeutic exploration might lead to some general psychologic benefits, such as greater acceptance or understanding of her relationships with her family. Of course, dynamic formulations can sometimes be seductive, facile explanations for a more complex reality. They should not be treated as absolute truth, but simply as a guiding construct—a way of organizing experience. Nevertheless, it may be that some premorbid risk factors such as abuse or neglect, more than any identifiable disorder, are significantly associated with the subsequent development of CFS.

Our immediate focus has been on trying to relieve her suffering and maintain and possibly increase her level of functioning. We know that the illness has interfered with her work, her care of the home, her marriage, her relationships with her kids, her finances, her planning, and her mobility. Depression appears to have been a secondary problem, and sleep disturbance, pain, counterproductive overexertion, financial pressure, marital conflict resulting from the illness, and insufficient social support have all been identified as important problems to ameliorate. These issues provide a sufficient focus for psychologic intervention and support.

For some symptoms, such as cognitive impairment, neuropsychologic testing may be helpful in documenting the areas of difficulty and suggesting compensatory strategies. The range of neuropsychiatric symptoms experienced by "Janice" was striking, and was perhaps the most persuasive evidence for the presence of an organic process. As further evidence, two electroencephalograms showed mild abnormalities in the temporal area and nerve conduction studies revealed the presence of a mild peripheral neuropathy. Further brain imaging procedures such as SPECT or BEAM might be useful, but they also might generate false-positive findings. These procedures are still relatively new, and their high sensitivity can identify subtle changes the significance of which is unknown.

The bottom line is that for "Janice" or any other patient with CFS, it is important to form an alliance around the patient's perception of the illness and, at the same time, to keep an open mind about a range of alternative hypotheses.

CONCLUSION

Patients with complaints of chronic fatigue have an increased prevalence of psychiatric disorders, especially depression, organic mental syndromes, and panic disorder. The prevalence of premorbid psychiatric disorders among patients who meet criteria for CFS is unclear. Several studies have indicated a higher prevalence, although some studies have not. Aside from sampling differences in the groups studied, there are major methodologic difficulties in applying *DSM III-R* definitions of affective and somatoform disorders in patients with prominent physical symptoms. Differences in interpretation of these definitions may account for a major degree of the discrepancy. In the future it would be wiser to follow the lead of those who have used measurements of depression, and other psychiatric disorders, specifically modified for physically ill patients. One also has to suspend the CDC criterion that requires no history of psychiatric disorders if one hopes to resolve the issue of pre-morbid psychopathology in CFS.

Although the evidence is not entirely clear, much of the increase in psychiatric disorder among patients with CFS appears to be secondary to the development of the syndrome. This is especially true for the cognitive dysfunction and depression. The prevalence of depression, although far higher than in the general population, is only slightly higher in CFS than in other chronic medical conditions involving fatigue as a prominent symptom. In all these disorders, the severity of fatigue correlates highly with the degree of depression.

The psychologic impact of CFS is enormous. The challenge to these patients' sense of validity and credibility, the uncertainty and unpredictability of the disorder, and the frequent cognitive difficulties are particularly difficult features of the syndrome with which to cope. Psychiatric treatment can have an important adjunctive role, provided that it is presented to patients in an acceptable way and not as an alternative to medical care. The physician's role is to rule out other causes for the chronic fatigue, to use empirical treatments to alleviate symptoms, and to facilitate an adequate support system for the patient.

REFERENCES

1. Holmes, G.P., Kaplan, J.E., Gantz, N.M., et al. Chronic fatigue syndrome: A working case definition. *Ann. Intern. Med.* 108:387, 1988.
2. Myalgic encephalomyelitis by proxy. *Br. Med. J.* 299:1030, 1989.
3. Manu, P., Lane, T.J., and Matthews, D.A. The frequency of chronic fatigue syndrome in patients with symptoms of persistent fatigue. *Ann. Intern. Med.* 109:554, 1988.
4. Manu, P., Matthews, D.A., and Lane, T.J. The mental health of patients with a chief complaint of chronic fatigue syndrome: A prospective evaluation and follow-up. *Arch. Intern. Med.* 148:2213, 1988.
5. Manu, P., Matthews, D.A., and Lane T.J. Panic disorder among patients with chronic fatigue. *South. Med. J.* 84:451, 1991.
6. Katon, W.J., Buchwald, D.S., Simon, G.E., et al. Psychiatric illness in patients with chronic fatigue and those with rheumatoid arthritis. *J. Gen. Intern. Med.* 6:277, 1991.
7. Kruesi, M.J., Dale, J., and Straus, S.E. Psychiatric diagnoses in patients who have chronic fatigue syndrome. *J. Clin. Psychiatry* 50:53, 1989.

8. Krupp, L.B., Friedberg, F., Fernquist, S., et al. Chronic fatigue syndrome and psychological symptoms. Proceedings of the Annual Meeting of the Society of Behavioral Medicine 14:34, 1990.
9. Hickie, I., Lloyd, A., Wakefield, D., and Parker, G. The psychiatric status of patients with the chronic fatigue syndrome. *Br. J. Psychiatry* 156:534, 1990.
10. Powell, R., Dolan, R., and Wessely, S. Attributions and self-esteem in depression and chronic fatigue syndromes. *J. Psychosom. Res.* 34:665, 1990.
11. Wessely, S., and Powell, R. Fatigue syndromes: a comparison of chronic "postviral" fatigue with neuromuscular and affective disorders. *J. Neurol. Neurosurg. Psychiatry* 52:940, 1989.
12. Altay, H.T., Toner, B.B., Brooker, H., et al. The neuropsychological dimensions of postinfectious neuromyasthenia (chronic fatigue syndrome): A preliminary report. *Int. J. Psychiatry Med.* 20:141, 1990.
13. Bastien, S. Patterns of Neuropsychological abnormalities and cognitive impairment in adults and children. Presented at the Cambridge Symposium on Myalgic Encephalitis, Cambridge University, England, April 1990.
14. Daugherty, S.A., Henry, B.E., Peterson, D.L., et al. Chronic fatigue syndrome in northern Nevada. *Rev. Infect. Dis.* 13 (Suppl.):S39, 1991.
15. Sandman, C. Is there a CFS dementia? *CFIDS Chronicle*, Spring Conference Issue, 1991. p. 105.
16. Becker, J.T. Methodologic considerations in assessment of cognitive function in chronic fatigue syndrome. *Rev. Infect. Dis.* 13 (Suppl.):S112, 1991.
17. Cohen-Cole, S.A., and Stoudemire, A. Major depression and physical illness: Special considerations in diagnosis and biological treatment. *Psychiatr. Clin. North Am.* 10:1, 1987.
18. Abbey, S.E., Toner, B.B., Garfinkel, P.E., et al. Self-report symptoms that predict major depression in patients with prominent physical symptoms. *Int. J. Psychiatry Med.* 20:247, 1990.
19. Krupp, L.B., Mendelson, W.B., and Friedman, R. An overview of chronic fatigue syndrome. *J. Clin. Psychiatry* 52:403, 1991.
20. Abbey, S.E., and Garfinkel, P.E. Neurasthenia and chronic fatigue syndrome: The role of culture in the making of a diagnosis. *Am. J. Psychiatry* 148:1638, 1991.
21. Straus, S.E., Tosato, G., Armstrong, G., et al. Persisting illness and fatigue in adults with evidence of EBV infection. *Ann. Intern. Med.* 102:7, 1985.
22. McEvedy, C.P., and Beard, A.W. A controlled follow-up of cases involved in an epidemic of "benign myalgic encephalomyelitis." *Br. J. Psychiatry* 77:1376, 1973.
23. Wessely, S. Mass hysteria: Two syndromes? *Psychol. Med.* 17:109, 1987.
24. Greenberg, D. Neurasthenia in the 1980s: Chronic mononucleosis, chronic fatigue syndrome, and anxiety and depressive disorders. *Psychosomatics* 31:129, 1990.
25. Moldofsky, H. Nonrestorative sleep and symptoms after a febrile illness in patients with fibrositis or chronic fatigue syndromes. *J. Rheumatol.* 19 (Suppl.):150, 1989.
26. Krupp, L.B., Mendelson, W.B. Sleep in chronic fatigue syndrome. *Sleep* (Suppl.):261, 1991.
27. Demitrack, M.A., Dale, J.K., Straus, S.E., et al. Evidence for impaired activation of the hypothalamic–pituitary–adrenal axis in patients with chronic fatigue syndrome. *J. Clin. Endocrinol. Metab.* 73:1224, 1991.
28. English, T.L. Skeptical of skeptics. *J.A.M.A.* 265:964, 1991.
29. Kansky, G. Cartoon. The Massachusetts CFIDS Update, Winter 1990. Pp. 9, 10.
30. Buchwald, D., Sullivan, J.L., Komaroff, A.L. Frequency of chronic active

Epstein-Barr virus infection in a general medical practice. *J.A.M.A.* 257:2303, 1987.

31. Onischenko, T.G. Cognitive rehabilitation: Strategies, tasks, theories, and games. *CFIDS Chronicle* 1:7, 1991.
32. Mena, I. Study of cerebral perfusion by neuro SPECT in patients with chronic fatigue syndrome. Presented at Chronic Fatigue Syndrome and Fibromyalgia: Pathogenesis and Treatment, First International Conference, Los Angeles, February 1990.
33. Buchwald, D., Cheney, P.R., Peterson, D.L., et al. A chronic illness characterized by fatigue, neurologic and immunologic disorders, and active human herpesvirus type 6 infection. *Ann. Intern. Med.* 116:103, 1992.
34. Goldstein, J. Functional brain imaging in CFIDS. *CFIDS Chronicle*, Spring Conference Issue, 1991, p. 101.
35. Parker, J.C., Frank, R.G., Beck, N.C., et al. Pain management in rheumatoid arthritis patients: A cognitive behavioral approach. *Arthritis Rheum.* 31:593, 1988.
36. Spiegel, D., Kraemer, H.C., Bloom, J.R., and Gottheil, E. Effect of psychosocial treatment on survival of patients with metastatic breast cancer. *Lancet* 2:888, 1989.
37. Wessely, S., David, A., Butler, S., et al. Management of chronic (post-viral) fatigue syndrome. *J. R. Coll. Gen. Pract.* 39:26, 1989.
38. Butler, S., Chalder, T., Ron, M., and Wesseley, S. Cognitive behavior therapy in chronic fatigue syndrome. *J. Neurol. Neurosurg. Psychiatry* 54:153, 1991.
39. Gracious, B., Wisner, K.L. Nortriptyline in chronic fatigue syndrome: A double-blind, placebo-controlled single case study. *Biol. Psychiatry* 15:405, 1990.
40. Goodnick, P.J. Bupropion in chronic fatigue syndrome. *Am. J. Psychiatry* 147:1091, 1990.
41. Goodnick, P.J., Extein, I. Bupropion and fluoxetine in depressive subtypes. *Ann. Clin. Psychiatry* 1:119, 1989.
42. Canadian Cooperative Multiple Sclerosis Study: A randomized controlled clinical trial of amantadine in fatigue associated with multiple sclerosis. *Can. J. Neurol. Sci.* 14:273, 1987.
43. Krupp, L.B., Coyle, P.K., Cross, A.H., et al. Amelioration of fatigue in multiple sclerosis patients with pemoline. *Ann. Neurol.* 26:155, 1989.

4

Richard B. Schwartz

Neuroradiologic Features

Chronic fatigue syndrome (CFS) is associated with a variety of neurologic signs and symptoms including headache, impaired cognitive abilities, and disturbances in sensory and motor functions. The neuroradiologic findings in CFS are less well documented. There have been only two reports of radiologic abnormalities in CFS, both analyzing the same patient population from an outbreak in northern Nevada in the mid-1980s. Daugherty and co-workers [1] studied magnetic resonance (MR) images in 15 patients and found abnormalities on all scans; Buchwald et al. [2] noted MR abnormalities in 79% of 142 patients. In both studies, the most common finding was foci of increased T_2 signal in the centrum semiovale and periventricular or subcortical white matter. Occasionally, these zones of increased signal were confluent. Buchwald et al. noted that when signal abnormalities were located in the occipital radiations, internal capsule or cerebellar white matter, the location of the lesion tended to correlate with symptomatology. Furthermore, in those patients in whom serial MR scans were obtained, MR abnormalities persisted despite improvements in the patient's condition.

At the Brigham and Women's Hospital, we have studied 32 patients with CFS. Single-photon emission computed tomography (SPECT) was performed in all subjects, and MR in 16. The abnormalities on MR examination were similar in appearance to those noted by Buchwald and Daugherty and their colleagues, the most frequent findings being small foci of increased T_2 signal in the white matter (Fig. 4-1) that occasionally

69

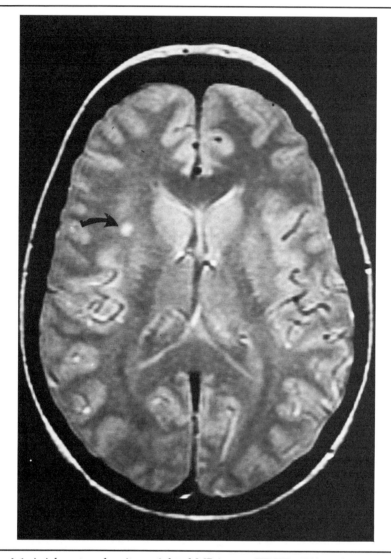

Fig. 4-1. Axial proton density-weighted MR image (TR/TE: 4000 ms/20 ms) shows a single focus of increased signal in the subcortical right frontal white matter *(arrow)*. Note that the focus is of brighter signal than the adjacent cerebrospinal fluid.

appeared confluent (Fig. 4-2). However, we noted that MR abnormalities were present in only approximately 60% of the subjects. Abnormalities on SPECT occurred with greater frequency, although not all subjects had abnormalities on both examinations. When abnormalities were present on both studies, the findings on SPECT appeared to be more extensive and to correlate better with the severity of disease than did MR.

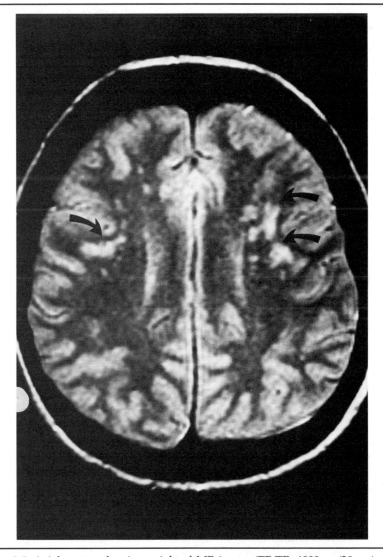

Fig. 4-2. Axial proton density-weighted MR image (TR/TE: 4000 ms/20 ms) shows regions of confluent increased signal in the centrum semiovale bilaterally *(arrows)*.

MR FINDINGS

Foci of increased T_2 signal on MR are not specific for CFS, and in fact may be seen in a variety of conditions [3–9]. Similar abnormalities have been reported in ischemic disease (lacunar infarcts or subcortical arteriosclerotic encephalopathy), multiple sclerosis, vasculitis (systemic lupus erythematosus, Behçet's disease, or other autoimmune diseases), viral infection or postviral demyelination, exposure to toxic agents, radiation changes, and even migraine [7,8]. Furthermore, prominence of the Virchow-Robin perivascular spaces is noted in normal individuals (état criblé). The clinical history is sufficient to exclude the majority of conditions that may mimic the findings of CFS; the most important distinction to make radiologically is between CFS and multiple sclerosis, focal ischemia, or normal perivascular spaces.

Multiple Sclerosis

Multiple sclerosis is manifested radiographically by T_2-bright foci in a periventricular distribution, representing demyelination. Since these lesions follow the course of cortical venules, they tend to be ovoid and abut the ependymal lining. They often coalesce, involving large white matter tracts such as the corpus callosum and middle cerebellar peduncles; the location of such lesions is virtually pathognomonic for multiple sclerosis. In patients whose scans show only a few small foci of increased signal, however, it may be difficult to distinguish this pattern from CFS.

Focal Ischemia

Ischemic lesions caused by small vessel disease are typified by foci of increased T_2 signal in the centrum semiovale and periventricular regions, where they are usually separated from the ventricular wall by at least a centimeter; this pattern is similar to that seen in CFS. However, this form of ischemic white matter disease increases with age, and is uncommon in the population usually affected by CFS. Vasculitis is one cause of focal ischemic abnormalities that occurs independent of age, but often small cortical lesions are present on MR as well, a feature that has not been noted in CFS.

Normal Perivascular Spaces

The distribution of the lesions seen on MR images in CFS is similar to that seen in état criblé, a benign asymptomatic condition of unknown cause in which prominent perivascular (Virchow-Robin) spaces are noted radiographically and pathologically. However, this radiographic appearance is much more common in patients with CFS than in the general population; it was observed in 79% of patients with CFS but only 21% of healthy controls, according to Buchwald et al. In addition, when present, the T_2-bright foci appear to be more numerous in CFS patients than in normal subjects. More importantly, true benign Virchow-Robin perivascular spaces are filled with cerebrospinal fluid, and therefore should follow the signal characteristics of fluid in the ventricular system. In CFS, however, these spaces tend to have abnormally increased T_2 signal, suggesting an abnormality of the fluid within them or the neuropil surrounding them. This finding is consistent with either or both a perivascular cellular infiltrate caused by viral infection or demyelination of the surrounding white matter from an immune complex mediated response to the infection [2].

SPECT FINDINGS

On SPECT, multiple foci of decreased perfusion are present that appear to be more extensive than the MR abnormalities and tend to involve both white and gray matter; the cortex is normal on MR. The cause of the cortical involvement measured by SPECT is unclear, but possible explanations include the retrograde effects of demyelination on cell bodies (wallerian degeneration), direct infection of neuroglial elements, or occlusion of small arterioles and arteries from an inflammatory process (vasculitis).

CONCLUSION

Information concerning the neuroradiologic findings in CFS is meager. The available data indicate that the syndrome is associated with a pattern of foci or confluent areas of increased white matter T_2 signal on MR. These findings are nonspecific and poorly understood, but are believed to reflect the effects of a viral illness on the central nervous system. The radiographic findings represent either cellular infiltration of the perivascular spaces, focal demyelination in response to the infection, or disease involving the small vessels of the cerebral white matter. SPECT has shown an extensive pattern of decreased perfusion that may more accurately reflect the severity of the disease.

Ongoing studies in our institution include precise mapping of MR and SPECT abnormalities, longitudinal studies, and correlation of radiographic abnormalities with clinical information. These efforts may help us to establish more accurately the diagnosis and prognosis in individual cases of CFS, and ultimately to understand more fully the pathogenesis of the syndrome.

REFERENCES

1. Daugherty, S.A., Henry, B.E., Peterson, D.L., et al. Chronic fatigue syndrome in northern Nevada. *Rev. Infect. Dis.* 13 (Suppl.): S31, 1991.
2. Buchwald, D., Cheney, P.R., Peterson, D.L., et al. A chronic illness characterized by fatigue, neurologic and immunologic disorders, and active human herpesvirus-6 infection. *Ann. Intern. Med.* 116:102, 1992.
3. Jungreis, C.A., Kanak, E., Hirsch, W.L., et al. Normal perivascular spaces mimicking lacunar infarction. *Radiology* 169:101, 1988.
4. Sze, G., De Armond, S.J., Brant-Zawadzki, M., et al. Foci of MRI signal (pseudolesions) anterior to the frontal horns: Histological correlations of a normal finding. *A.J.N.R.* 7:381, 1986.
5. Zimmerman, R.D., Fleming, C.A., Lee, B.C.P., et al. Periventricular hyperintensity as seen by magnetic resonance: Prevalence and significance. *A.J.R.* 146:443, 1986.
6. Kirkpatrick, J.B., and Hayman, L.A. White-matter lesions in MR imaging of

clinically healthy brains of elderly subjects: Possible pathologic basis. *Radiology* 162:509, 1987.
7. Masters, J.J. Ischemia, hydrocephalus, atrophy and neurodegenerative disorders: MRI experience at high field strength in S.J. Pomeranz (ed.), *Craniospinal Magnetic Resonance Imaging.*Philadelphia, Saunders, 1989.
8. Wallace, C.J., Seland, T.P., Fong, T.C. Multiple sclerosis: The impact of MR imaging. *A.J.R.* 158:849, 1992.
9. Sewell, K.L., Livneh, A., Aranow, C.B., and Gravzel, A.I. Magnetic resonance imaging versus computed tomographic scanning in neuropsychiatric systemic lupus erythematosus. *Am. J. Med.* 86:625, 1989.

5

Don L. Goldenberg

Fibromyalgia Syndrome and Its Overlap with Chronic Fatigue Syndrome

Chronic fatigue is a prominent symptom in systemic connective tissue disorders such as rheumatoid arthritis (RA) and systemic lupus erythematosus. During the past decade, rheumatologists have become interested in another chronic musculoskeletal pain condition associated with chronic fatigue. This condition, previously termed fibrositis and now called *fibromyalgia*, is—like the chronic fatigue syndrome (CFS)—a syndrome rather than a specific disease, at least at this formative stage of its development. The purpose of this chapter is to review the clinical characteristics and diagnostic criteria of fibromyalgia, discuss the clinical features that overlap with CFS, and describe potential pathophysiologic and therapeutic similarities of fibromyalgia and CFS.

HISTORICAL PERSPECTIVE

The syndrome of fibromyalgia was clearly delineated in the French literature in the 1850s. The term *fibrositis,* coined by Sir William Gowers in 1904, became popular at the turn of the century following pathologic descriptions of "inflammation" in muscle biopsies from patients thought to have the disorder [1]. Investigators were unable to replicate these findings, however, and the disorder fell out of mainstream academic interest during most of the twentieth century. Nevertheless, many physicians continued to be interested in the concept of local muscle pain

75

without discrete structural changes. Kellgren injected saline into muscles and demonstrated a reproducible pattern of referred pain [2]. Physiatrists such as Janet Travell popularized the concept of muscle "trigger points" within the framework of myofascial pain syndrome [3].

Fibrositis, as it was usually called, often became a wastebasket term for any poorly understood chronic pain disorder. Since there were no reproducible findings on physical examination or laboratory testing, physicians often viewed fibromyalgia as a form of "psychogenic rheumatism." Just as epidemic CFS was often thought to be an example of "mass hysteria," so was fibromyalgia considered to be "all in the head."

CLINICAL CHARACTERISTICS AND DIAGNOSTIC CRITERIA

Fibromyalgia and CFS are both ultimately diagnoses of exclusion. The concept of such a syndrome is best applied when more discrete illnesses such as RA, systemic lupus erythematosus, or Lyme disease have been excluded. Nevertheless, the clinical features of fibromyalgia are characteristic and diagnostic criteria have been established.

The cardinal symptom is chronic, generalized pain. Fatigue is present in 80 to 90% of patients. Other prominent symptoms include sleep disturbances, stiffness, paresthesias, depression or anxiety, headache, and irritable bowel syndrome [4]. The pain is reported to be of high intensity, generally more severe than the pain of RA [5]. Patients with fibromyalgia also report that the pain is more radiating than that of RA, and use more adjectives when describing their pain.

The musculoskeletal examination is unremarkable aside from tenderness at discrete anatomic locations (Fig. 5-1). These "tender points" are also widespread and usually bilaterally symmetric. They tend to cluster in areas that are commonly tender in regional soft tissue pain disorders, such as the neck and shoulders, lateral epicondyle, second costochondral junction, low back, and outer, lateral hip. Small joints commonly tender in RA are infrequently tender in fibromyalgia. A number of potential tender point schema were reported to distinguish fibromyalgia patients from normal controls and patients with other musculoskeletal pain conditions [4].

The diagnosis of fibromyalgia (or, for that matter, CFS) should be considered in any patient with chronic, unexplained, generalized musculoskeletal pain. Most patients have had symptoms for years and have generally undergone multiple, inconclusive diagnostic tests. Patients usually look well and the physical examination is unremarkable other than the presence of the tender points. The examiner should palpate for tenderness with manual pressure approximating 4 kg at specific locations (see Fig. 5-1). The amount of pressure needed to elicit pain at these locations should be compared to control locations such as the

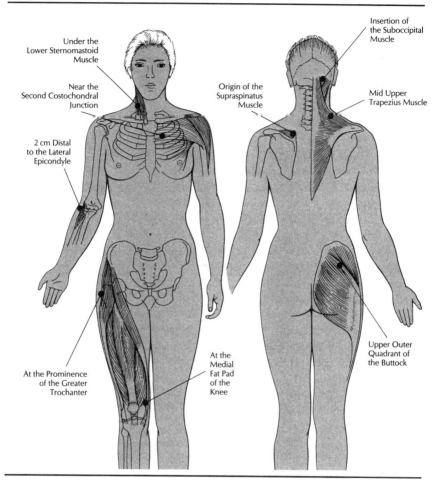

Fig. 5-1. Tenderness at characteristic musculoskeletal locations establishes fibromyalgia as a consistent entity. The nine "tender points" depicted are important in diagnosis: Each is bilateral, for a total of 18 test sites widely distributed on the body surface, and tenderness on digital palpation of at least 11 in a patient with at least a 3-month history of diffuse musculoskeletal pain is recommended as the diagnostic standard for fibromyalgia. (Reproduced with permission. From D. L. Goldenberg: Diagnostic and Therapeutic Challenges of Fibromyalgia. *Hosp. Practice* 24:9A.P.45.)

midfoot or the forehead. Tenderness is most marked at these specific locations, but patients with fibromyalgia show more tenderness than healthy controls at most locations [6]. In clinical investigations, it has been helpful to measure the tenderness more precisely using a dolorimeter or algometer, spring-loaded gauges that quantitate the amount of pressure.

In 1990, the American College of Rheumatology published criteria for the classification of fibromyalgia [7]. Investigators from 16 medical cen-

Table 5-1. Diagnostic criteria for fibromyalgia compared to those for chronic fatigue syndrome

Fibromyalgia	Chronic fatigue syndrome
Generalized pain, including axial, upper and lower extremities, and bilateral, for at least 3 months	Major: New onset of persistent, severe fatigue and exclusion of systemic illness
At least 11 of 18 tender points	Minor: Headache, sleep disorder, neuropsychiatric symptoms, myalgias, arthralgias, sore throat, painful lymphadenopathy, low-grade fever, pharyngitis

ters in North America compared 293 patients with fibromyalgia to 265 patients with rheumatic disorders most likely to cause problems in differential diagnosis, such as idiopathic low back pain. "Secondary" fibromyalgia patients were matched to controls with the corresponding "primary" rheumatic illness, such as RA. Each patient was administered a standard history, a physical examination including manual and dolorimeter examination of tender points by a blinded assessor, as well as appropriate laboratory tests. Multiple possible combinations of symptoms and signs were evaluated for optimal sensitivity and specificity in distinguishing patients with fibromyalgia from controls. The criteria selected were: (1) generalized pain, which must be present for at least 3 months and be located above and below the waist, at the right and left side, as well as the axial region; and (2) excessive tenderness on palpation of at least 11 of the 18 tender point sites depicted in Figure 5-1. This combination provided for a sensitivity of 88% and specificity of 81% in differentiating fibromyalgia from rheumatic disease controls. In terms of classification criteria, there was no utility to the concept of primary and secondary fibromyalgia. No exclusionary or inclusionary laboratory or radiologic tests were recommended for classification of fibromyalgia.

These and previous classification criteria for fibromyalgia have been extensively tested against appropriate controls, in contrast to the initial CDC working case definition for CFS. The CFS criteria do, however, describe many of the clinical features typical of fibromyalgia. It is not surprising that the suggested diagnostic criteria for fibromylagia and CFS are similar (Table 5-1) since the two conditions share so many clinical features. Both occur most often in women aged 20 to 50, although there is a greater female predominance in fibromyalgia, 8 or 10 to 1. Chronic fatigue is present in virtually all fibromyalgia patients, as mentioned, and myalgias occur in 90% of CFS patients. Other symptoms present in the majority of patients with both conditions include headache, neurocognitive and psychologic symptoms, and sleep disturbances.

Table 5-2. Clinical and tender point comparison of patients with fibromyalgia and chronic fatigue syndrome[a]

	Fibromyalgia (N = 20)[b]	CFS with musculoskeletal pain (N = 19)[b]	CFS without musculoskeletal pain (N = 8)
Mean age (yr)	42 ± 10.9	37 ± 11.6	36 ± 15.3
Duration of symptoms (mo)	84 ± 27.8	59 ± 33.4	51 ± 28.9
Fatigue	18 (90)	19 (100)	8 (100)
Sleep disturbance	19 (90)	18 (95)	6 (75)
Morning stiffness	19 (95)	12 (63)	5 (63)
Irritable bowel syndrome	16 (80)	10 (53)	5 (63)
Numbness and tingling	17 (85)	13 (68)	4 (50)
Raynaud's phenomenon	2 (10)[c]	7 (37)	4 (50)
Currently seeing mental health professional	2 (10)[c]	11 (58)	4 (50)
Past psychiatric disorder	5 (25)	4 (21)	2 (25)
Current psychiatric disorder	7 (35)	6 (32)	3 (38)
No. of tender points (manual examination)	19 ± 4.2	14 ± 6.7	6.4 ± 5.4[c]
Mean dolorimeter tender point score (kg/cm^2)	3.6 ± 1.4	3.8 ± 1.2	5.8 ± 1.6[c]

[a]Where appropriate, data are mean ± SD.
[b]Data are number (percent) of patients except as noted.
[c]$P \leq 0.05$, fibromyalgia versus CFS patients.
Source: From D. L. Goldenberg et al. [9].

CLINICAL SIMILARITIES BETWEEN FIBROMYALGIA AND CFS

During the past few years, we have reported two studies on the overlapping clinical features of fibromyalgia and CFS. In the first, 50 consecutive fibromyalgia patients were given a questionnaire used by our colleagues for the diagnosis of CFS [8]. The presence and severity of fatigue in these patients was similar to that in CFS, as was the presence of myalgias and neuropsychologic symptoms. More surprising, fibromyalgia patients frequently reported recurrent sore throat and low-grade fevers, and 55% reported that their symptoms began with a viral or flulike illness. There was no difference in mean antibody levels against Epstein-Barr virus (EBV) in the two groups, and neither differed from those of normal controls.

In the second study we examined 27 patients with CFS, 20 with fibromyalgia, and 10 normal controls [9]. All were age-matched women. In addition to a history and standard physical examination, each patient and control underwent a manual and dolorimeter tender point examination. The clinical characteristics of the fibromyalgia and CFS patients were nearly identical (Table 5-2). Eight of the 27 CFS patients did not complain of myalgias, and their mean results on manual and dolorimeter tender point examination were similar to the values in normal controls. In contrast, the tender point examination of the 19 CFS patients with myalgias was similar to that of the fibromyalgia patients. Thus, 19 of the 27 CFS patients met the diagnostic criteria for fibromyalgia.

PATHOPHYSIOLOGIC SIMILARITIES BETWEEN FIBROMYALGIA AND CFS

Infectious and Immunologic Mechanisms

Not only are the clinical manifestations of fibromyalgia and CFS strikingly similar, so too are the potential pathophysiologic mechanisms that have been investigated. CFS historically has been thought to be of infectious origin, although no single agent has ever been conclusively linked with the syndrome. Indeed, many CFS investigators a priori insist that the diagnosis of CFS be restricted to patients whose illness developed after a typical infection. This concept has not been tested, however, and we do not know whether flulike symptoms are more common at the onset of CFS than in other medical conditions.

Epidemics described with the term benign myalgic encephalomyelitis (BME) or epidemic neuromyasthenia were reported from many countries from 1930 through 1960. In 1985, two independent studies linked EBV to CFS [10]. However, case-control studies failed to demonstrate a difference in EBV antibodies in CFS and controls, and elevated antibodies to multiple viruses were often present in CFS. Enteroviruses, especially Coxsackie B, were higher in BME than in controls and were more often isolated from stool specimens [11]. Enteroviral RNA has been found in about 25% of CFS muscle biopsies but not in controls. Antibodies to human T cell leukemia virus and possible sequences of the viral genome have been reported more often in CFS than in controls. Other viruses recently studied in CFS include herpes simplex, cytomegalovirus, human herpesvirus 6, and "spuma virus."

Until recently, there has never been a similar focus on a possible infectious origin for fibromyalgia. Because more than 50% of our fibromyalgia patients reported that their condition began with a flulike illness [8], it is not surprising that investigators are now more often citing an association of fibromyalgia with a specific infection. Sigal reported that 25 of the first 100 patients referred to a Lyme disease center had fibromyalgia, including 17 with previous and 3 with current Lyme disease [12]. None of the fibromyalgia patients responded to antibiotics used to treat Lyme disease. Fibromyalgia has also been reported in association with human immunodeficiency virus [13], coxsackievirus [14], and parvovirus [15].

CFS investigations have often focused on immunologic abnormalities, especially those typical of a chronic viral illness. Although decreased total gamma globulin or gamma globulin subsets, T cell dysfunction, abnormal cellular immunity, and natural killer (NK) cell dysfunction have been reported in CFS, the abnormalities do not occur in the majority of patients, vary greatly in individual studies, and do not correlate with clinical symptoms. Most importantly, profound immune dysregulation and opportunistic infections have not been reported in CFS. Similar, nonspecific immune dysfunction has been reported in fibromyalgia [16].

Muscle Disease

Fibromyalgia has most often been considered to be a consequence of muscle disease. Nevertheless, inflammation or other altered muscle structure has not been prominent and in general has not differed from that of appropriate control muscle biopsies [17]. Studies of muscle strength, nerve conduction, and fatigability have also provided variable results. Recent studies of muscle in fibromyalgia and CFS have searched for evidence of excessive intracellular acidosis using techniques such as oxygen probe, chemical analysis of biopsied tissue, or nuclear magnetic resonance spectroscopy [18]. Such studies have indeed demonstrated evidence for excess muscle cell acidosis. However, these changes could be simply the result of pain and physical deconditioning. Patients with fibromyalgia have been found to be deconditioned, and a cardiovascular fitness training program can improve their symptoms [19]. Investigations of muscle function and physiology must control patients levels of physical fitness in future studies of fibromyalgia and CFS.

Neuropsychiatric Abnormalities

The findings on neuropsychiatric studies in fibromyalgia and CFS also are similar. This is especially true with regard to studies of depression. In most reports of fibromyalgia and CFS, the prevalence of major depression has ranged from 25 to 50%—percentages well above that of normal patients and higher than in other chronic illnesses such as RA. We found a 25% prevalence of current major depression in our fibromyalgia patients but a 70% lifetime history of major depression [20]. These numbers were both higher than for RA controls. Generally the depression antedated fibromyalgia by years. Similarly, most reports in CFS have cited a high premorbid history of depression. Wessely and Powell found depression in 47% of CFS patients including 43% with a premorbid psychiatric history [21]. Katon et al. found a 15% current and 76% lifetime history of major depression in CFS compared to 3% and 42% respectively for RA [22]. This study noted a moderate increase in anxiety disorder and somatization in CFS compared to controls, as we reported for fibromyalgia.

The role of stress, helplessness, and heightened somatic concern in fibromyalgia and CFS is starting to be explored. Certainly, conditions

Table 5-3. Location of neurologic symptoms at the initial visit (N = 135)

Location	No. (%)
Bilateral UE & LE	44 (33)
Bilateral UE	38 (28)
Bilateral LE	9 (7)
Unilateral UE	15 (11)
Unilateral LE	6 (4)
Diffuse	6 (4)
Unspecified	17 (13)
Total	135 (100)

UE = upper extremity; LE = lower extremity.
Source: From R. W. Simms and D. L. Goldenberg [27].

such as these, in which a diagnosis is usually delayed for years while patients see multiple physicians and undergo a large battery of tests, would promote increased frustration, helplessness, and hypervigilance regarding one's health. Fibromyalgia patients were found to have more psychologic and life stress than those with RA [23]. Robbins et al. reported that fibromyalgia patients had greater somatic distress and illness worry than RA patients [24]. Wessely emphasized the discordance of the public and medicine's views of CFS and the effect this could have on outcome [25]. He also reported that 86% of CFS patients attributed their illness only to physical cause. This "external attribution" of illness may impair the ability of CFS patients to become independent and take greater responsibility for treatment of their condition.

Other neuropsychiatric studies besides those emphasizing mood disorders have been reported more commonly in CFS. These especially have investigated the sensory and cognitive disturbances often reported in the syndrome. Prasher et al. found that auditory brainstem, median nerve somatosensory, and pattern-reversal checkerboard visual potentials were normal in 37 CFS patients, but attention deficits and slower speed of information processing were reported in some [26]. Preliminary reports of tiny white dots on magnetic resonance scans in a significantly greater number of CFS patients than controls need to be confirmed.

Neurologic Abnormalities

Paresthesias are common in both fibromyalgia and CFS, but a standard neurologic examination, nerve conduction studies, and electromyograms do not generally provide an explanation for their presence [27]. In fibromyalgia, we found that more than 80% of patients complained of numbness, tingling, or burning in an extremity (Table 5-3). These "neuropathic" symptoms often led to further invasive diagnostic tests (Table 5-4) and sometimes unnecessary surgery.

Table 5-4. Neurodiagnostic evaluation before diagnosis of fibromyalgia
(N = 54)

Test	No. performed	Result
Electromyography/nerve conduction velocity	36	32 normal, 2 positive for CTS,[a] 1 equivocal for CTS,[b] 1 not available
Myelography	1	Normal in all
CT scans (4 brain, 7 lumbar, 4 C-spine)	15	8 normal, 2 DJD C-spine, 2 DJD L-spine, 3 "disk space narrowing" at L4–5
Magnetic resonance imaging	4	Normal in all
Visual evoked potentials	1	Normal

[a]Median nerve motor latency > 4.5 msec.
[b]Median motor latency = 4.5 msec.
CTS = carpal tunnel syndrome, DJD = degenerative joint disease.
Source: From R. W. Simms and D. L. Goldenberg [27].

Sleep disturbances have been reported commonly in fibromyalgia and CFS. Moldofsky was the first to report an abnormal stage IV sleep pattern, described as alpha-delta sleep, in fibromyalgia [28]. He more recently reported a similar sleep electroencephalographic pattern in CFS [29]. However, other sleep disturbances, such as nocturnal myoclonus and sleep apnea, have been reported in patients with fibromyalgia. Furthermore, these sleep disturbances are reported in many disorders nad have been linked with fatigue in patients with RA [30].

Etiologic Possibilities in Fibromyalgia and CFS

A plausible unifying hypothesis in both fibromyalgia and CFS integrates the central and peripheral nervous system (Fig. 5-2). Any number of traumatic conditions, including an acute or chronic infection, could initiate a cascade of events that would promote a nociceptive disorder, fatigue, sleep disturbances, and depression. The immune system may act as a regulatory mechanism in this cascade. For example, sleep is under the influence of cytokines and neurotransmitters [31]. Immune abnormalities have been reported in depression, including altered cellular immune function and decreased NK cell activity [32]. In particular, the interaction of severe life stress and major depression produced a 50% reduction of NK cytotoxicity. Glaser et al. demonstrated that first year medical students during the time of examinations had a significant decrease in interferon as well as evidence of reactivation of EBV [33]. These immune changes correlated with the students' self-reported alterations in the state of their health.

The increased premorbid prevalence of depression in fibromyalgia and CFS could be considered a predisposing factor to chronic illness following the "stress" of an acute infection or psychologic stress. This

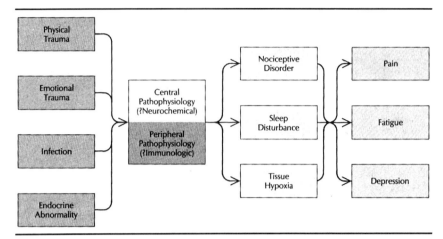

Fig. 5-2. Hypothetical origin of fibromyalgia. (Reproduced with permission. From D. L. Goldenberg: Diagnostic and therapeutic challenges of fibromyalgia. *Hosp. Practice* 24:9A.P.49. Illustration by Albert Miller.)

Table 5-5. Premorbid psychologic status of patients with normal or prolonged convalescence following Asian influenza of 1957

	Median test result	
Premorbid psychologic test	*Normal convalescence* (N = 14)	*Prolonged convalescence* (N = 12)
Total Cornell Medical Index (CMI) score	9.0	16.0[a]
Psychologic score on CMI	1.3	3.5[a]
Depression subscale on MMPI	51.5	61.0[a]

[a]Significant (P = 0.05) differences in the two groups.
MMPI = Minnesota Multiphasic Personality Inventory.
Source: Modified from J. B. Imboden, A. Canter, and L. E. Cluff [34].

hypothesis has previously been investigated. For example, Imboden et al. noted that convalescence from acute brucellosis and influenza correlated with the patient's preexisting emotional state [34]. In a fascinating prospective study of 600 military personnel prior to the 1957 Asian influenza epidemic, patients who had a prolonged (> 21 days) convalescence differed from those who were asymptomatic after 2 weeks only based on their premorbid psychologic status, particularly regarding measures of depression (Table 5-5).

Neuroendocrine Abnormalities in Fibromyalgia

Abnormal nociception has been proposed as a central factor in fibromyalgia. Heightened pain perception has been demonstrated at tender point sites as well as at control anatomic regions. Exaggerated response to pressure or to electrical pulse is present over normal and tender muscles [35]. Furthermore, excessive wheal and flare local skin reactions can be demonstrated after skin pressure or application of a chemical irritant such as capsaicin [36]. Abnormal peripheral vasospasm producing a Raynaud-like exaggerated response to cold is present in 40% of fibromyalgia patients and was found to correlate with serotonergic receptors [37].

More basic investigations of the afferent (sensory) and efferent (sympathetic) peripheral nervous system and interactions with the immune system are being reported in fibromyalgia. Substance P, a neurotransmitter important in pain transmission, was found to be elevated in the cerebrospinal fluid of patients with the disorder [38]. Musculoskeletal symptoms suggestive of fibromyalgia were reported in carcinoid syndrome, and improved after treatment with a somatostatin analog [39]. The hyperalgesia of fibromyalgia resembles that of neurologic conditions believed to involve the sympathetic nervous system, such as reflex sympathetic dystrophy. Extremity pain in fibromyalgia improved following a sympathetic block [40].

The complicated bidirectional interaction of the immune and nervous systems is of great interest. Substances such as beta-endorphins, enkephalins, and serotonin influence both systems. Levels of neurotransmitters have recently been measured in the plasma and cerebrospinal fluid of patients with fibromyalgia and, although the results are preliminary and not uniform, such measures should provide a fertile area of research. An abnormal neuroendocrine response, including the hypothalamic-pituitary-adrenal axis, has been reported in a subset of fibromyalgia patients [41].

THERAPY AND PROGNOSIS

Treatment for fibromyalgia and CFS has been based on different principles. Fibromyalgia has been approached as a chronic inflammatory condition, whereas therapy for CFS has largely focused on its possible infectious or immune origin. Unfortunately, no single treatment approach has been highly effective in the majority of patients.

In fibromyalgia, a number of randomized, controlled therapeutic trials have demonstrated that low doses of tricyclic medication, in particular amitriptyline and cyclobenzaprine, were more effective than placebo [42]. In contrast, nonsteroidal anti-inflammatory medications (NSAIDs) such as naproxen or ibuprofen, or even modest doses of prednisone, were no better than placebo. Combination therapy consisting of a central nervous system (CNS) active agent and an NSAID may be most effective. Two combinations tested have been amitriptyline with naproxen and ibuprofen with alprazolam [42,43]. The mode of action of tricyclics in low doses, such as 10 to 50 mg at bedtime, may involve their effect on

Table 5-6. Therapeutic principles for fibromyalgia and chronic fatigue syndrome

Education:
What syndrome "is" and "is not"
The mind-body interaction
Emphasize independence
Medication:
Treat sleep disturbance
Analgesia
Activity-exercise program:
Appropriate rest-activity cycle
Gentle cardiovascular fitness training
"Hands-on" physical therapy, massage, etc.
Longitudinal support:
Counseling
Relaxation, cognitive-behavior therapy

neurotransmitters, which may lessen sleep disturbances as well as alter pain perception. Other medications reported to have some benefit in fibromyalgia include 5-hydroxytryptophan and a compound containing carisoprodol and acetaminophen. Nonmedicinal treatments found to be effective in controlled clinical trials in fibromyalgia include cardiovascular fitness training, electromyographic (EMG) biofeedback, hypnotherapy, and cognitive-behavior training. However, longitudinal studies of patients with fibromyalgia show that few enter remission, most continue to have at least moderate levels of pain, and many note a major impact on their function in the workplace [44].

Controlled clinical trials in CFS include acyclovir, immune globulin, and ampligen (see Chapter 14). Acyclovir was no better than placebo and the two studies of gamma globulin demonstrated no or only slight benefit, but the preliminary results of the ampligen trial appear encouraging. In uncontrolled reports, CNS-active medications and cognitive-behavior therapy have also been reported to be of some benefit in CFS. Long-term longitudinal studies have not been reported in CFS.

I would propose that treatment follow similar principles at this "formative" stage of development of the syndromes currently termed fibromyalgia and CFS (Table 5-6). The foundation of treatment should be education of the patient and family about the condition. An explanation of what the condition "is" should include how the diagnosis is made and why these disorders are so controversial with reassurance that the condition is not "all in the head." Equal emphasis on what it "is not" should focus on the fact that these disorders are not life-threatening, disfiguring, or degenerative. An explanation of the complicated interaction of mind and body will provide the patient with a basis for understanding the role of stress, depression, and anxiety on pain and fatigue. Such an understanding will also promote the patient's sense of independence in treating these disorders.

Until specific medications have been proved highly effective in the majority of patients, symptoms such as sleep disturbances and pain should be treated with agents such as tricyclics in low doses and simple analgesics. If major depression or anxiety is present, it should be treated with effective doses of psychopharmacologic medications.

An activity and exercise program should be initiated in slow increments. This should include avoidance of prolonged bed rest and moderation of physically or emotionally stressful situations. A carefully controlled, low-impact cardiovascular fitness training program should be started that includes activities such as walking, biking, or water exercises. "Hands-on" physical therapy or modalities such as massage, deep tissue manipulation, ultrasound, heat, cold, electrical stimulation, and acupuncture may be helpful, although no controlled therapeutic trials have been reported.

A team approach to ambulatory management of patients with these syndromes can best integrate the various aspects of education, physical and exercise therapy, medication, and counseling. Formal behavior modification such as cognitive-behavior and relaxation response training are effective methods to improve coping with chronic medical illness. For example, patients must not view themselves as the victims of some unknown infection but recognize that, as with any chronic illness, they can help to determine how they respond to treatment.

An emerging important and controversial aspect of these syndromes involves disability and medicolegal issues. Considerable attention has been given to these issues in fibromyalgia, for which in the United States approximately 15% of patients have received disability payments whereas in Sweden, with national health insurance, 40% of patients receive disability pay for the disorder. This is despite the fact that in fibromyalgia, as well as in CFS, it is impossible to document cause or degrees of disability objectively on physical examination or through usual laboratory or radiologic testing. A patient's self-assessment of pain, fatigue, and other symptoms is the major factor determining work capacity. Nevertheless, fibromyalgia and CFS patients in the United States have been granted disability benefits, especially from the Social Security Administration, although legal battles often had to be fought.

CONCLUSION

Fibromyalgia is a common clinical syndrome of chronic musculoskeletal pain. There is no evidence of joint or muscle inflammation, and the presence of tenderness at discrete anatomic locations is the only uniform finding on physical examination. Nearly all patients with fibromyalgia have chronic, marked fatigue, and indeed, the clinical features of fibromyalgia and CFS are strikingly similar. The two syndromes share many pathogenetic features as well.

It is especially important for neurologists to be keenly aware of these disorders in view of the significant neuropsychiatric symptoms. These include paresthesias, cognitive deficits, and psychologic symptoms. Patients are often referred to neurologists, and the differential diagnosis may include multiple sclerosis, peripheral neuropathy, entrapment disorders such as carpal tunnel syndrome, radiculopathies, or major depression. Neurologists are also uniquely trained to evaluate and treat such patients since they are used to caring for patients with chronic illness and with myopathic and neuropathic symptoms, and to dealing with the psychosocial aspects of debilitating disorders. Neurologists are also best equipped to play a major role in future basic research to better understand these two frustrating syndromes.

REFERENCES

1. Gowers, W.R. Lumbago: Its lessons and analogues. *Br. Med. J.* 1:117, 1904.
2. Kellgren, J.H. Observations of referred pain arising from muscle. *Clin. Sci.* 3:175, 1938.
3. Travell, J., and Simons, D.G. *Myofascial Pain and Dysfunction: The Trigger Point Manual,* Baltimore: Williams & Willkins, 1983.
4. Goldenberg, D.L. Fibromyalgia syndrome: An emerging but controversial condition. *J.A.M.A.* 257:2782, 1987.
5. Leavitt, F., Katz, R.S., Golden, H.E., et al. Comparison of pain properties in fibromyalgia patients and rheumatoid arthritis patients. *Arthritis Rheum.* 29:775, 1986.
6. Simms, R.W., Goldenberg, D.L., Felson, D.T., and Mason, J.H. Tenderness in 75 anatomic sites: Distinguishing fibromyalgia patients from controls. *Arthritis Rheum.* 31:182, 1988.
7. Wolfe, F., Smythe, H.A., Yunus, M.B., et al. The American College of Rheumatology 1990 Criteria for the Classification of Fibromyalgia: Report of the Multicenter Criteria Committee. *Arthritis Rheum.* 33:160, 1990.
8. Buchwald, D., Goldenberg, D.L., Sullivan, J.L. and Komaroff, A.L. The "chronic, active Epstein-Barr virus infection" syndrome and primary fibromyalgia. *Arthritis Rheum.* 30:1132, 1987.
9. Goldenberg, D.L., Simms, R.W., Geiger, A., and Komaroff, A.L. High frequency of fibromyalgia in patients with chronic fatigue seen in a primary care practice. *Arthritis Rheum.* 33:381, 1990.
10. Komaroff, A.L., and Goldenberg, D. The chronic fatigue syndrome: Definition, current studies and lessons for fibromyalgia research. *J. Rheumatol.* 19 (Suppl.):23, 1989.
11. Behan, P.O., Behan, W.M.H., and Bell, E.J. The postviral fatigue syndrome—An analysis of the findings in 50 cases. *J. Infect.* 10:211, 1985.
12. Sigal, L.H. Summary of the first 100 patients seen at a Lyme disease referral center. *Am. J. Med.* 88:577, 1990.
13. Buskila, D., Gladman, D.D., Langevitz, P., et al. Fibromyalgia in human immunodeficiency virus infection. *J. Rheumatol.* 17:1202, 1990.
14. Nash, P., Chard, M., and Hazleman, B. Chronic Coxsackie B infection mimicking primary fibromyalgia. *J. Rheumatol.* 16:1506, 1989.
15. Leventhal, L.J., Naides, S.J., and Freundlich, B. Fibromyalgia and parvovirus infection. *Arthritis Rheum.* 34:1325, 1991.

16. Wallace, D.J., Bowman, R.L., Wormsley, S.B., and Peter, J.B. Cytokines and immune regulation in patients with fibrositis. *Arthritis Rheum.* 32:1334, 1989.
17. Yunus, M.B., and Kalyan-Raman, U.P. Muscle biopsy findings in primary fibromyalgia and other forms of nonarticular rheumatism. *Rheum. Dis. Clin. North Am.* 15:115, 1989.
18. Bennett, R.M. Muscle physiology and cold reactivity in the fibromyalgia syndrome. *Rheum. Dis. Clin. North Am.* 15:135, 1989.
19. McCain, G.A., Bell, D.A., Mai, F.M., and Halliday, P.D. A controlled study of the effects of a supervised cardiovascular fitness training program on the manifestations of fibromyalgia. *Arthritis Rheum.* 31:1135, 1988.
20. Goldenberg, D.L. Psychologic studies in fibrositis. *Am. J. Med.* 81:67, 1986.
21. Wessely, S., and Powell, R. Fatigue syndromes: A comparison of chronic "postviral" fatigue with neuromuscular and affective disorders. *J. Neurol. Neurosurg. Psychiatry* 52:940, 1989.
22. Katon, W.J., Buchwald, D.S., Simon, G.E., et al. Psychiatric illness in patients with chronic fatigue and those with rheumatoid arthritis. *J. Gen. Intern. Med.* 6:277, 1991.
23. Uveges, J.M., Parker, J.C., Smarr, K.L., et al. Psychological symptoms in primary fibromyalgia syndrome: Relationship to pain, life stress, and sleep disturbance. *Arthritis Rheum.* 33:1279, 1990.
24. Robbins, J.M., Kirmayer, L.J., and Kapusta, M.A. Illness worry and disability in fibromyalgia syndrome. *Int. J. Psychiatry Med.* 20:49, 1990.
25. Wessely, S. Old wine in new bottles: Neurasthenia and "ME." *Psychol. Med.* 20:35, 1990.
26. Prasher, D., Smith, A., Findley, L. Sensory and cognitive event-related potentials in myalgic encephalomyelitis. *J. Neurol. Neurosurg. Psychiatry* 53:247, 1990.
27. Simms, R.W., and Goldenberg, D.L. Symptoms mimicking neurologic disorders in fibromyalgia syndrome. *J. Rheumatol.* 15:1271, 1988.
28. Moldofsky, H. Rheumatic pain modulation syndrome: The interrelationships between sleep, central nervous system serotonin, and pain. *Adv. Neurol.* 33:51, 1982.
29. Moldofsky, H. Nonrestorative sleep and symptoms after a febrile illness in patients with fibrositis and chronic fatigue syndromes. *J. Rheumatol.* 19 (Suppl.):150, 1989.
30. Mahowald, M.W., Mahowald, M.L., Bundle, S.R., and Ytterberg, S.R. Sleep fragmentation in rheumatoid arthritis. *Arthritis Rheum.* 32:974, 1989.
31. Krueger, J.M., and Johannsen, L. Bacterial products, cytokines and sleep. *J. Rheumatol.* 19 (Suppl.):52, 1989.
32. Irwin, M., Patterson, T., Smith, T.L., et al. Reduction of immune function in life stress and depression. *Biol. Psychiatry* 27:22, 1990.
33. Glaser, R., Rice, J., Sheridan, J., et al. Stress-related immune suppression: Health implications. *Brain Behav. Immun.* 1:7, 1987.
34. Imboden, J.B., Canter, A., and Cluff, L.E. Convalescence from influenza. *Arch. Intern. Med.* 108:393, 1961.
35. Scudds, R.A., Trachsel, L.C., Luckhurst, B.J., and Percy, J.S. A comparative study of pain, sleep quality and pain responsiveness in fibrositis and myofascial pain syndrome. *J. Rheumatol.* 19 (Suppl.):120, 1989.
36. Littlejohn, G.O., Weinstein, C., and Helme, R.D. Increased neurogenic inflammation in fibrositis syndrome. *J. Rheumatol.* 14:1022, 1987.
37. Bennett, R.M., Clark, S.R., Campbell, S.M., et al. Symptoms of Raynaud's syndrome in patients with fibromyalgia—A study utilizing the Nielsen test, digital photoplethysmography, and measurements of platelet alpha$_2$-adrenergic receptors. *Arthritis Rheum.* 34:264, 1991.

38. Vaeroy, H., Helle, R., Forre, O., et al. Elevated CFS levels of substance P and high incidence of Raynaud phenomenon in patients with fibromyalgia: New features for diagnosis. *Pain* 32:21, 1988.
39. Smith, S., Anthony, L., Roberts, L.J., et al. Resolution of musculoskeletal symptoms in the carcinoid syndrome after treatment with the somatostatin analog octreotide. *Ann. Intern. Med.* 112:66, 1990.
40. Bengtsson, A., and Bengtsson, M. Regional sympathetic blockade in primary fibromyalgia. *Pain* 33:161, 1988.
41. McCain, G.A., and Tilbe, K.S. Diurnal hormone variation in fibromyalgia syndrome: A comparison with rheumatoid arthritis. *J. Rheumatol.* 19 (Suppl.):154, 1989.
42. Goldenberg, D.L., Felson, D.T., and Dinerman, H. A randomized, controlled trial of amitriptyline and naproxen in the treatment of patients with fibromyalgia. *Arthritis Rheum.* 29:1371, 1986.
43. Russell, I.J., Fletcher, E.M., Michalek, J.E., et al. Treatment of primary fibrositis/fibromyalgia syndrome with ibuprofen and alprazolam—A double-blind, placebo-controlled study. *Arthritis Rheum.* 34:552, 1991.
44. Felson, D.T., and Goldenberg, D.L. The natural history of fibromyalgia. *Arthritis Rheum.* 29:1522, 1986.

Heather M. A. Cavanagh
John W. Gow
Kathleen Simpson
Lindsay J. A. Morrison
Wilhelmina M. H. Behan
Peter O. Behan

6

Special Aspects of Virology

The chronic fatigue syndrome (CFS), also known as chronic fatigue and immune dysfunction syndrome (CFIDS) in the United States, is a disease of unknown origin. It is poorly defined with the diagnosis tending to be made on the basis of overwhelming fatigue for which no other cause can be found. A similar but better characterized disorder is the postviral fatigue syndrome (PFS), which starts abruptly following an apparent viral infection. No specific etiologic agent has been found in these fatigue syndromes, although a variety of viruses have been implicated. Well-documented outbreaks have followed infection by Coxsackie [1], polio [2], Epstein-Barr [3], and rubella or varicella [4] viruses. Retroviruses have also been associated with the syndrome [5].

One of the many problems encountered in the search for an infectious agent in CFS is the lack of positive serologic findings. Numerous studies have been carried out but, because of the ubiquitous viruses believed to be involved, it has proved very difficult to identify any differences between patients and the general population. Several investigators have reported that the incidence of increased antibody titers against enteroviruses or Epstein-Barr virus (EBV) is greater in patients with CFS than in controls [6,7], but such data cannot be accepted unless they are based on careful epidemiologic studies. The serologic findings have therefore been used mainly to indicate which viruses warrant further investigation and to investigate any possible role for immune dysfunction in this syndrome.

THE ENTEROVIRUS THEORY

Epidemics have occurred worldwide since the first report of the disorder, at the Los Angeles County Hospital in 1934 [2,8–13]. This initial outbreak was followed by a major epidemic in Akureyri, Iceland [14]. The spread within the community, with 5% of the male and 8% of the female population affected, pointed to an infectious agent but all attempts at isolation proved negative. Five years later, however, a widespread outbreak of poliomyelitis due to type 1 virus occurred in Iceland affecting all areas except those where Akureyri disease (CFS) had occurred [15]. Serologic studies suggested that the CFS patients, immune to poliomyelitis, had already been exposed to an agent immunologically similar, but not identical, to the poliomyelitis virus. An additional observation, again suggestive of the involvement of an infectious agent, was that when an American airman who had caught poliomyelitis in the 1955 Iceland epidemic returned to his home town of Pittsfield, Massachusetts, a small outbreak of CFS followed [16,17].

In successive years, epidemics continued to be reported and their nature continued to suggest that an infectious agent, although not detected, must be responsible, with a probable incubation period of between 8 and 10 days, perhaps reaching 3 to 4 weeks in some outbreaks. The mode of transmission was unknown but personal contact appeared probable. In most cases an acute illness resulted that lasted a few weeks, but in others the syndrome persisted for months or even years.

An outbreak that occurred between 1980 and 1983 in Scotland appeared to suggest that Coxsackie virus might be the agent. Serologic studies revealed that 82% of the patients had increased titers of neutralizing antibody to Coxsackie B virus antibodies compared to 10% of the control population [18]. This led to widespread interest in the role of Coxsackie viruses, or enteroviruses in general, in CFS. Detection of the viral structural protein antigen VP1 in 56% of patients compared to no controls, with 89% of the former group still positive 4 months later, added to the evidence pointing to enteroviruses as a causative agent of CFS [19].

Evidence from Molecular Biology Studies

The application of molecular biology techniques has led to evidence of the persistence of enteroviral sequences in the muscle of a proportion of CFS patients. Two main molecular biology techniques have been used, molecular hybridization and the polymerase chain reaction (PCR) [20]. Molecular hybridization utilizes the fact that complementary strands of

DNA (cDNA), or RNA, will anneal under certain conditions. Thus, by using a radiolabeled probe specific for enteroviruses, patient RNA or DNA samples can be examined for the presence of enteroviral genomes and visualized by autoradiography. However, stringent controls must be adhered to. Strands of DNA or RNA that are only partially similar will anneal under nonstringent conditions. In addition, it is not unknown for viral sequences to be similar enough to certain small regions of human genomic sequences to allow at least limited annealing. The probe must therefore be carefully chosen and stringently tested for nonspecific binding to human sequences.

PCR is a highly sensitive alternative technique that can also be used in the detection of viral genomes in patient RNA or DNA. This technique is dependent upon the annealing of two small fragments of single-stranded DNA to the specific target sequence (e.g., an enteroviral genome within the patient sample). Copies of the target sequence are then synthesized in vitro and products can be analyzed by agarose gel electrophoresis or by molecular hybridization. This technique in effect amplifies, up to 10^6-fold, any specific target sequences within the patient sample. It is this amplification of starting material which makes PCR such a highly sensitive technique, allowing detection of viral sequences present at lower concentrations than would be detectable by molecular hybridization.

PCR is not without drawbacks, however. The technique is so sensitive that the smallest level of contamination will lead to false-positive results. Again, as with molecular hybridization, it is not unknown for PCR primers to amplify nontarget genomic sequences. Extreme care must therefore be taken to keep all instruments and solutions clean and contamination free. Confirmation of the specificity of amplified sequence should routinely be carried out by determining the DNA sequence of the amplified fragment in addition to routine molecular hybridization.

Archard et al. [21] demonstrated the presence of enteroviral sequences in the muscle of CFS patients using molecular probes. Quantitative slot-blot hybridization was utilized with a cloned Coxsackie virus cDNA probe complementary to the highly conserved RNA-dependent RNA polymerase coding region of the viral genome. The probe was confirmed as enterovirus group specific by hybridization to RNA purified from cells infected with a range of enteroviral serotypes. Twenty-four percent of muscle biopsies from patients with CFS were found to contain enteroviral sequences compared with none from the controls. This was believed to be a conservative estimate of positive findings because of the probable focal nature of any persistent enteroviral infection in muscle and the small amount of tissue available in the biopsy [22].

Gow et al. [23,24] then applied the more sensitive PCR technique, using primers to the highly conserved 5' nontranslated region (NTR) of the viral genome, to look for copies of the enteroviral genome in peripheral blood leukocytes and muscle of CFS patients (Fig. 6-1). The PCR

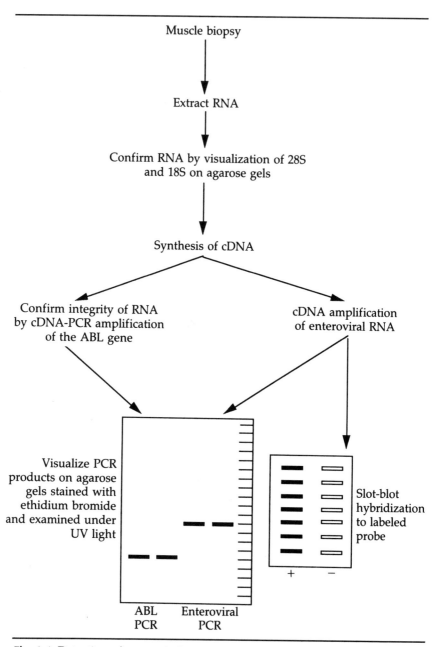

Fig. 6-1. Detection of enteroviral sequences by PCR

results confirmed the presence of enteroviral sequences in the muscle of CFS patients: 53% of patients were positive compared to 15% of controls. (*Note:* The positive control cases all had neoplasia, carcinoma of either the breast or the colon.) With regard to the leukocyte samples,

PCR results showed that 16% of both patients and controls were positive: it was therefore of great interest that patients were 3.5 times more likely to demonstrate the presence of enteroviral sequences in their muscle.

Studies of Viral Persistence

The mechanism of enteroviral persistence is unclear. Previous studies have suggested that defective replication of the viral genome is responsible for persistence. In a normal enteroviral cytolytic infection, the synthesis of plus strands (genomic or sense strands) to minus strands (template or antisense strands) occurs in a ratio of approximately 100 : 1. This asymmetric synthesis of the plus and minus strands reflects the requirement for each strand in the life cycle of the virus. The plus strand encodes all the viral proteins, both enzymatic and structural, and is packaged into the completed capsid to be released from the infected cell and continue the infectious cycle. The minus strand, however, has only one function: to act as a template for the preferential production of plus strand RNA.

Molecular Hybridization Experiments
Cunningham et al. [25] attempted to determine the relative levels of genomic and template RNA in muscle from patients with CFS. Riboprobe vectors were constructed that contained the RNA-dependent, RNA polymerase coding region of the Coxsackie virus genome in both orientations. Probes complementary to the positive and negative strand could then be synthesized independently. RNA was prepared from muscle biopsies from patients and probed with both the complementary plus and the complementary minus strand from the riboprobe vector. By using equal amounts of RNA from each patient and equal amounts of probe for each slot-blot, the results could be used to indicate the relative amount of each strand present within the RNA sample; this is because the plus strand from the riboprobe hybridizes only to the minus strand of the virus, and the minus strand from the riboprobe hybridizes only to any plus strand viral RNA in the sample. This technique was used to demonstrate that samples from 4 CFS patients, which were positive for enterovirus RNA, contained similar amounts of the plus and minus strands; i.e., the ratio of plus to minus strands was now 1 : 1 instead of the 100 : 1 ratio seen in usual cytolytic infection.

PCR Experiments
Recent data contradict the findings from the hybridization experiments. A novel method has been developed utilizing the more sensitive and specific PCR technique to determine the ratio of plus to minus strands in RNA samples from similar patients. The protocol is shown schematically in Figure 6-2 [26]. The ability of PCR to enhance the quantity of each strand present in the RNA samples from patients is exploited by

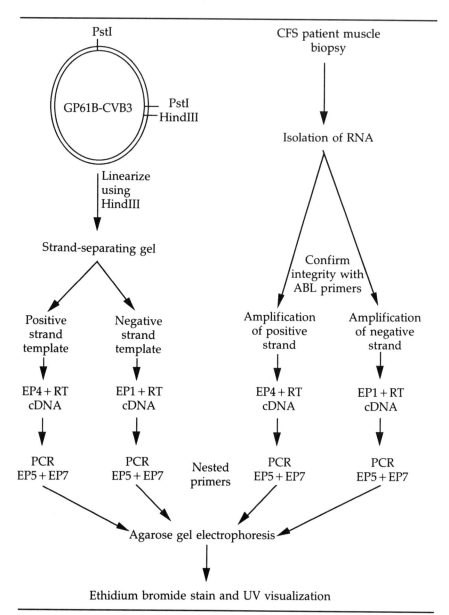

Fig. 6-2. A novel technique developed for detection of single strands of RNA. Plasmid GP61B-CVB3 DNA is utilized as a positive control. Synthesis of each strand of the plasmid DNA should be equal in each experiment. Synthesis of cDNA in the absence of reverse transcriptase (RT) is negligible in all cases. (From J.W. Gow, et al. Replication of enteroviruses in muscle from postviral fatigue syndrome patients. *J. Cell. Biochem.* 16(c):142, 1992. Copyright © 1992. Reprinted by permission of Wiley-Liss, a division of John Wiley and Sons, Inc.)

synthesizing cDNA copies of either the plus or the minus strand. A single 26bp primer (EP4) complementary to the plus strand is used in conjunction with reverse transcriptase to specifically synthesize single-stranded cDNA copies of that strand. Nested primers (EP5 and EP7) are then used to synthesize double-stranded cDNA PCR fragments from the sample. The amount of single-stranded cDNA in the initial reaction should be directly proportional to the amount of plus strand RNA in the original starting material. Therefore, amplification of the single-stranded cDNA by the nested primers will still be proportional to the initial amount of plus strand RNA. The technique is carried out simultaneously using a 26bp primer (EP1) complementary to the minus strand to synthesize the initial single-stranded cDNA.

The technique was shown to be quantitative by utilizing a plasmid containing 530bp of the Coxsackie virus B3 (CVB3) 5′ NTR. The vector was linearized using restriction endonucleases. Single-stranded DNA was then obtained by electrophoresing the plasmid through a strand-separating agarose gel. Purified single strands were put through the described procedure in the presence or absence of reverse transcriptase to ensure that any amplification was not due simply to priming of the original plasmid DNA. Using this control procedure, it could be demonstrated that both strands were copied in equal amounts during the PCR reaction, as would be expected, since equal amounts of plasmid DNA were used in each reaction. Priming from the original plasmid DNA in the absence of reverse transcriptase was negligible.

When the technique was applied to samples from patients with CFS, the ratio of plus strands to minus strands was demonstrated to be in the region of 100 : 1. The results of one experiment are shown in Figure 6-3. Thus, it appears that the replication ability of the persistent enteroviral genomes in this muscle is normal, at least at the level of transcription. Sequence mutation resulting in abnormal protein production or structure may, however, play a role.

Molecular Evidence for Persistent Enteroviruses

This information may prove central to the whole question of persistent enterovirus in CFS. If enterovirus persists, what is the mechanism? If a mutant virus is deficient in its replication, then why does it not simply cease to exist? If, however, the virus can replicate normally, then why do we not see an acute infection and why can the virus not be isolated by growth in tissue culture? Another factor to be considered is the role of immune dysfunction or deficiency of the host in the maintenance of viral persistence. Further research into the replicative ability of these persistent viruses, maintenance of persistence, and a detailed examination of the host response is required to elucidate the molecular basis of the pathogenetic role of these viruses in CFS, if any.

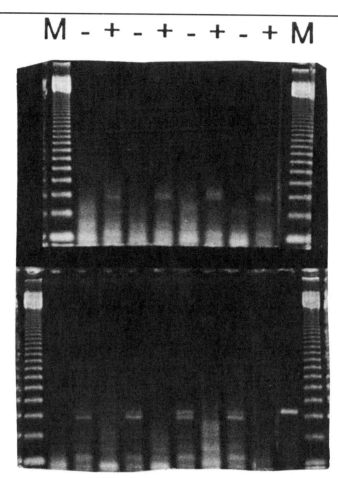

Fig. 6-3. Amplification of single strands of enteroviral RNA. RNA from muscle biopsies of CFS patients, known to contain enteroviral RNA, was analyzed by the procedure described in Fig. 6-2, to evaluate the ratio of plus strand to minus strand enteroviral RNA present. Each − and + pair represents amplification of either the minus (−) or plus (+) strand of enteroviral RNA from a single patient. The pair at lower right represents amplification of Coxsackie virus RNA, isolated from HeLa cells in culture, to demonstrate the ratio of plus to minus strand occuring in normal lytic infections (100 : 1). The ratio of plus strands to minus strands in the muscle of patients with CFS would appear to be approximately 100 : 1.

THE HERPESVIRUS THEORY

Epstein-Barr virus (infectious mononucleosis/glandular fever), varicella zoster virus (chickenpox), and cytomegalovirus have also been associated with CFS. Several studies have revealed that, following a herpesvirus infection, a minority of patients may go on to have chronic or recurrent symptoms for at least a year or longer [3,7,27–30].

Serologic evidence has indicated an active infection with EBV in 20% of CFS patients [31]. The majority of the population carry antibodies to EBV at any given time, but these "background" levels are purely indicative of past infection. However, 20% of CFS patients appear to demonstrate significantly raised titers of EBV specific early antigen (EA) antibodies. EA is expressed during the viral lytic cycle, and measurable anti-EA antibodies indicate increased production of the virus.

Molecular hybridization was again employed in the search for persistent EBV in CFS patients [32]. A cloned DNA probe unique to EBV but conserved between different isolates was utilized to detect the presence of the EBV genome in muscle biopsies from CFS patients. Nine percent of the patients examined (8 of 86) were positive for the presence of the EBV genome [33].

It is interesting to note that patients with raised antibody titers to EBV or persistence of EBV in muscle, as shown by molecular hybridization, were clearly distinct from those demonstrating an enteroviral infection. Patients with a persistent EBV infection were never positive for the presence of enterovirus, and those positive for persistent enteroviral infections were never demonstrated to have EBV.

THE ROLE OF RETROVIRUS IN CFS

The news that an HTLV-II-like retrovirus might be an etiologic agent in CFS [5] was received with great excitement. The idea of a retrovirus as a cause of CFS was attractive. A virus like HTLV-II could subtly disrupt the host immune system and allow other viruses to persist; it could also cause chronic release of cytokines, the toxic effect of which can mimic the symptoms of CFS. If such an exogenous retrovirus were involved in initiating the syndrome, then a diagnostic test could be quickly produced, to be of great benefit to patients and clinicians alike.

Evidence for a Retrovirus

The link between retroviruses and CFS was based on a study by De-Freitas et al. [5] of 30 patients with CFIDS, both adult and pediatric, with 13 exposure and 10 nonexposure controls. Exposure controls were defined as having had sexual or casual contact with CFS patients, whereas nonexposure controls claimed to have had no contact with any patients. DNA was obtained from patient and control blood samples and examined by PCR, Western blot, and in situ hybridization.

PCR primers were designed to amplify three regions: HTLV-I *gag*, HTLV-II *gag*, and HTLV-II *tax*. PCR products were electrophoresed in agarose gels and capillary blotted onto nylon filters. Internal oligonucleotide primers, end-labeled with ^{32}P, were then used as probes. No HTLV-I *gag*-like or HTLV-II *tax*-like sequences were detected in any sample. However, more than 75% of the patients showed HTLV-II *gag*-like sequences in their DNA compared with 34% of the exposure controls and none of the nonexposure controls.

Western immunoblotting was used to screen patient sera for the presence of HTLV antibodies. Western blotting is a technique that utilizes the binding of antibody to protein to analyze sera, cell lysates, and other constituents, for the presence of either specific proteins or specific antibodies. When patient sera were blotted against purified HTLV-I protein, more than 50% of the patients demonstrated antibodies to at least two viral gene products. Again, none of the nonexposure controls showed antibody against HTLV, whereas over 30% of exposure controls had antibodies to HTLV in their sera.

Finally, in situ hybridization was employed to determine whether the HTLV-II *gag* region amplified by PCR of patients' DNA was part of a functional gene. In situ hybridization uses the principles of molecular hybridization but is carried out on tissue sections or blood cells attached to slides or coverslips. Thus, by probing with radiolabeled DNA or RNA fragments, it is possible to use the procedure to detect either viral genomes or viral RNA transcripts. The presence of viral RNA transcripts (i.e., viral messenger RNA), reveals that active transcription of the viral genome is taking place within individual cells. Seven out of 10 HTLV-II *gag*-positive samples were shown by PCR to have cells expressing HTLV-II *gag* mRNA. The *gag*-positive cells were, however, rare (10^{-2} to 10^{-4}).

The investigators concluded that an association exists between this exogenous HTLV-II-like virus and CFS [5]. It has also been proposed that the CFS-related HTLV-II-like retrovirus is a member of the spumaretrovirus group, a "foamy" virus, closely related to HTLV-II (J. Martin, personal communication).

Evidence Against a Retrovirus

Again, controversy surrounds these results. As yet, no independent group has been able to duplicate the findings reported by DeFreitas and colleagues. Gow et al. [34] have used PCR to study 30 well-characterized patients who fulfilled the CDC exclusion criteria for CFS, all of whom were admitted as inpatients for detailed evaluation and had severe fatigue lasting more than a year. Thirty age- and sex-matched controls, including healthy volunteers and disease controls with autoimmune and muscle disorders, were also studied.

High-molecular-weight DNA was isolated from peripheral blood mononuclear cells. The fidelity of the DNA was assured by amplifying a 1 µg aliquot with endogenous tyrosine kinase control gene (ABL gene primers) [23]. Only those samples that gave a positive ABL gene band were used for analysis with the retroviral primers. Titration experiments

Table 6-1. Retroviral PCR amplification results[a]

PCR primers[b]	PCR results		Probe results	
	CFS	Controls		
HTLV-I/II *tax* SK43/44	Neg	Neg	ND	
HTLV-II *env* bp 5689–5713 6002–6026	Neg	Neg	ND	
HTLV-I/II *pol* SK110/111	Pos	Pos	SK112 SK118	neg neg
HTLV-II *gag* bp 1374–98 1573–97	Pos	Pos	pMT2	neg
HTLV-II *gag* bp 807–40[c] 1214–87[c]	Pos	Pos	pMT2 bp1080–1105[c]	neg neg

[a]Positive control/pMT2 (HTLV-I) DNA was positive for both sets of *gag* PCR primers and positive in subsequent hybridization with pMT2 and the bp1080–1105 *gag* probe. 30 CFS patients and 30 controls were studied.
[b]SK primers were obtained from Cetus.
[c]Primers as published in [5].
Neg = negative, pos = positive, ND = not done.

using an HTLV-II infected cell line serially diluted with uninfected cells confirmed that 1 infected target cell in approximately 100,000 uninfected cells could be detected. The results of amplification of DNA from patients and controls with a range of retroviral primers are shown in Table 6-1.

Experiments with *tax* and *env* primer were negative. *Pol* region primers gave rise to a product of approximately 186bp in both patients and controls, but this band did not hybridize to either HTLV-I or HTLV-II specific internal probes. *Gag* region primers gave rise to specific bands in all patients and controls. However, when the products were hybridized to retroviral sequences, no specific signal was detected. Hybridization of *gag* primer product with the internal *gag* probe [5] was also negative.

To investigate the claim that the virus present in CFS is an HTLV-II-related human foamy virus, a parallel study was performed on the serum of 20 CFS patients and 20 normal and disease controls [34]. Serum was examined by Western blot and indirect immunofluorescence (IFA). The Western blot and IFA results were negative for all patient and control samples.

Weighing the Evidence

Because one of these studies was carried out in the United States [5] and one in Europe [34], it has to be considered that an exogenous retrovirus might be present in the American but not in British patients. Even if this were the case, the virus could be opportunistic rather than the etiologic agent. Detection of exogenous retroviral sequences has been shown in the past to be controversial: for instance, previous reports of a possible retroviral agent in multiple sclerosis (MS) have now been discounted [35–37]. The initial detection of retroviral sequences in MS was shown to result from either contamination of the patient samples with positive control DNA or amplification of endogenous retroviral sequences.

We therefore must await conclusive evidence to substantiate the existence of an exogenous retrovirus, if any, in CFS.

THE POSSIBLE ROLE OF PERSISTENT VIRUS

Acute viral infections have traditionally attracted the most interest, but it has become apparent that numerous viruses (e.g., herpes simplex, cytomegalovirus, Epstein-Barr, rubella, and adenoviruses) can cause chronic viral disease [38]. A variety of clinical patterns can be produced by such chronic infections, and since the pattern depends on the host's response as well as the virus, the same agent can be responsible for more than one syndrome [39].

Chronic viral infections can be divided into two main groups: persistent, when infectious virus can be identified, and latent, when it cannot. Examples of persistent virus infection include those due to measles, rubella, the papova group, and some of the herpes group, while others of the herpes and retrovirus groups (e.g., herpes simplex and zoster) are associated with latency. In both types, infectious virions can be assembled and therefore the complete viral genome is present.

The main areas of interest with regard to a possible relationship between CFS and a chronic viral infection are, first, whether the disease could be produced by an as yet undetected virus, and second, how such a virus might cause the various symptoms and at the same time escape immune surveillance.

Characteristics of a Chronic Virus

In a chronic viral illness, the virus is limited in its effects but is not eliminated. At any given time, only a few cells are involved and any tissue damage is repaired. Infected cells may not be killed and may be able to reproduce, but they are unlikely to be able to carry out specialized functions [40]. One of the major conceptual advances in recent virology has been the realization that these viruses cause disease by destroying specialized functions in differentiated cells without killing them or interfering with their basic "housekeeping" functions. Oldstone et al [41,42] demonstrated this ability using an animal model of C3H/ST mice persistently infected with lymphocytic choriomeningitis virus (LCMV). In this mouse strain, LCMV preferentially infects growth hormone (GH) producing cells in the pituitary gland, but not prolactin-producing cells, and disrupts the synthesis of GH, leading to growth retardation and hypoglycemia in persistently infected mice. Despite this, the cells remain free of structural injury [43,44].

If the virus succeeds in evading the immune response, evidence of its presence will be difficult to detect. It may be impossible to isolate by the usual methods and may not show a cytopathic effect in any but a highly susceptible cell line, light and electron microscopy may not reveal viral particles, and immunostaining of infected cells will be negative if viral antigen is not expressed. In addition, the patient cannot be expected to show a rising titer of specific antibody, although a constant level of antibody against the infecting agent may be maintained.

The presence of a persistent virus may be causing several organic changes within the host. It is known that the symptoms of CFS may be mimicked by high levels of cytokines. Chronic release of these factors is known to induce fatigue, myalgia, headache, memory impairment, and sleep disturbance [15]. Could a persistent viral infection be responsible for such chronic release of cytokines in CFS? Studies investigating cytokine levels in CFS patients have proved conflicting and inconclusive [46]. Possible mechanisms for the cytokine theory are presented in Figure 6-4.

We have established an animal model that is being used in conjunction with patient analysis to determine the effects of persistent enteroviral infection in vivo. Initial results have indicated that interleukin-6 (IL-6) is unregulated in persistently infected mice. IL-6 has been shown to be produced in the central nervous system during viral infection [47] and continually secreted during persistent infection [48]. The relevance of these findings is being investigated.

Does Persistent Enterovirus Disrupt Calcium Transport?

Preliminary data from our laboratory suggest that abnormalities may exist in the intracellular Ca^{2+} transport pathways of some CFS patients. In addition, by utilizing DNA database search programs, we have identified an area of the enteroviral genome that demonstrates a high degree of similarity to regions of the cellular calcium-binding protein calsequestrin (CSQ) messenger RNA. The major role of CSQ, an acidic glycoprotein, is to buffer transported Ca^{2+} by serving as an intravesicular sink and thus to facilitate active transport. CSQ may also play an active role in the Ca^{2+} release mechanism [49,50]. It is conceivable that persistent enterovirus, which we have already demonstrated to be present in a high proportion of CFS patients, may be interfering with the CSQ-Ca^{2+} pathways and thereby causing the symptoms associated with CFS.

However, we have also noted this abnormality in other disorders

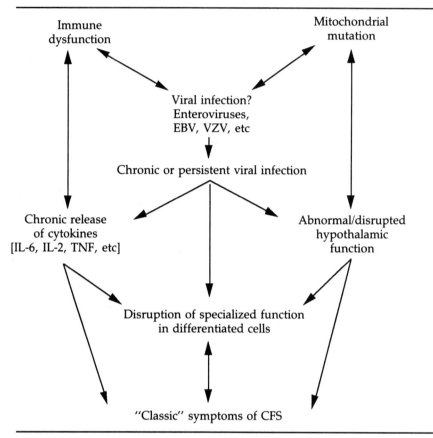

Fig. 6-4. Possible mechanisms of chronic fatigue syndrome

such as rheumatoid arthritis. It may be that the phenomenon occurs when a patient is inactive over long periods, or it may simply be associated with muscle fatigue in general. This phenomenon and its relationship to enteroviruses, if any, is being investigated.

CONCLUSION

When one reviews CFS with its epidemic and endemic data, clinical features, and laboratory results, it becomes clear that more questions than answers are available concerning the cause, or causes, of this intriguing syndrome. Conflicting evidence arises with regularity on every aspect of the disorder, from immunology to physiology and, not least, to viral involvement.

Viral agents have been strongly implicated by many groups, but as yet no single etiologic agent has been identified. Perhaps that one agent does not exist: We may have to revolutionize our thoughts to encompass the idea that several agents, viral and otherwise, or a combination thereof, are capable of inducing the same syndrome in conjunction with host susceptibility. The mechanism by which these factors trigger CFS may, however, be consistent throughout, irrespective of the etiologic agent. Thus, although several groups "support" several different viruses as causative agents, it may be that in the near future they will come together as supporters of a common mechanism, capable of induction by a variety of factors, rather than a single causative agent.

Alternatively, an unidentified, perhaps new virus may come to be recognized as the etiologic agent. Perhaps we are still looking at what are in fact secondary or opportunistic infections by EBV, enteroviruses, or other agents. The persistence of these viruses in the muscle of patients with CFS must, however, play an important role. It is most likely that, through finding the cause of this persistence, whether virally induced, host induced, or the result of a second virus, we may finally understand the cause of this debilitating syndrome.

REFERENCES

1. Stevenson, J., and Hambling, M. H. A case of Bornholm disease associated with Coxsackie virus group A type 9 infection. *Lancet* 2:873, 1971.
2. Gilliam, A. G. Epidemiological study of an epidemic, diagnosed as poliomyelitis, occurring among the personnel of the Los Angeles County General Hospital during the summer of 1934. U. S. Public Health Bulletin 240, Public Health Service. Washington, DC, US Government Printing Office, 1938. P. 90.
3. Hamblin, T. J., Hussain, J., Akbar, A. N., et al. Immunological reason for chronic ill health after infectious mononucleosis. *Br. Med. J.* 287:85, 1983.
4. Behan, P. O., Behan, W. M. H., and Bell, E. J. The postviral fatigue syndrome—An analysis of the findings in 50 cases. *J. Infect.* 10:211, 1985.
5. DeFreitas, E., Hilliard, B., Cheney, P. R. et al. Retroviral sequences related to human T-lymphotropic virus type II in patients with chronic fatigue immune dysfunction syndrome. *Proc. Natl. Acad. Sci. USA* 88:2922, 1991.
6. Calder, B. D., Warnock, P. J., McCartney, R. A., and Bell, E. J. Coxsackie B viruses and the postviral fatigue syndrome: A prospective study in general practice. *J. R. Coll. Gen. Pract.* 37:11, 1987.
7. Straus, S. E., Tosato, G., Armstrong, G., et al. Persisting illness and fatigue in adults with evidence of Epstein-Barr virus infection. *Ann. Intern. Med.* 102:7, 1985.
8. Marinacci, A. A., and von Hagen, K. D. The value of the electromyogram in the diagnosis of Iceland disease. *Electromyography* 5:241, 1965.
9. Stahel, H. Die Poliomyelitis—epidemie bei stab geb 1 R37 und Geb.Sch.Bat.11 Erstfeld, 18–30 Juli, 1937: Die Abortiv-Poliomyelitis. *Schweiz. Med. Wochen Achr.* 68:86, 1938.
10. Gsell, O. Abortive poliomyelitis. *Helv. Med. Acta* 16:169, 1949.
11. Gsell, O. Abortive poliomyelitis. Liepzig: Verlag Thieme, Chapter 13, 1938.
12. Houghton, L. E., and Jones, E. I. Persistent myalgia following a sore throat. *Lancet* 1:196, 1942.
13. McConnell, J. An epidemic of pleurodynia with prominent neurologic symptoms and no demonstrable cause. *Am. J. Med. Sci.* 209:41, 1945.

14. Sigurdsson, B., Sigurjonsson, J., Sigurdsson, J. H., et al. Disease epidemic in Iceland simulating poliomyelitis. *Am. J. Hyg.* 52:222, 1950.
15. Sigurdsson, B., Gudnadottir, M., and Petursson, G. Response to poliomyelitis vaccination. *Lancet* 1:370, 1958.
16. Henderson, D. A., and Shelekov, A. Epidemic neuromyasthenia: Clinical syndrome? *N. Engl. J. Med.* 260:757, 1959.
17. Hart, R. H. Epidemic neuromyasthenia. *N. Engl. J. Med.* 281:787, 1969.
18. Fegan, K. G., Behan, P. O., and Bell, E. J. Myalgic encephalomyelitis— Report of an epidemic. *J. R. Coll. Gen. Pract.* 33:335, 1983.
19. Yousef, G. E., Bell, E. J., Mann, G. F., et al. Chronic enterovirus infection in patients with postviral fatigue syndrome. *Lancet* 1:146, 1988.
20. Sambrook, J., Fritsch, E. F., and Maniatis, T. (eds.). *Molecular Cloning—A Laboratory Manual.* Cold Spring Harbor, N.Y.: Cold Spring Harbor Laboratory Press, 1989.
21. Archard, L. C., Behan, P. O., Bell, E. J., et al. Postviral fatigue syndrome: Persistence of enterovirus RNA in muscle and elevated creatine kinase. *J. R. Soc. Med.* 81:326, 1988.
22. Archard, L. C., Freeke, C. A., Richardson, P. J., et al. Persistence of enteroviral RNA in dilated cardiomyopathy: A progression from myocarditis. In Schultheis, H.-P. (ed.). *New Concepts in Viral Heart Disease.* Berlin: Springer-Verlag, 1988. Pp. 347–62.
23. Gow, J., Behan, W. M. H., Clements, G. B., et al. Enteroviral sequences detected by polymerase chain reaction in muscle biopsies of patients with postviral fatigue syndrome. *Br. Med. J.* 302:692, 1991.
24. Gow, J. W., and Behan, W. M. H. Amplification and identification of enteroviral sequences in the postviral fatigue syndrome. *Br. Med. Bull.* 47(4):872, 1991.
25. Cunningham, L., Bowles, N. E., Lane, R. J. M., et al. Persistence of enterovirus RNA in chronic fatigue syndrome is associated with the abnormal production of equal amounts of positive and negative strands of enteroviral RNA. *J. Gen. Virol.* 71:1399, 1990.
26. Gow, J. W., Simpson, K., Behan, W. M. H., Cavanagh, H. M. A., and Behan, P. O., Replication of enteroviruses in muscle from postviral fatigue syndrome patients. *J. Cell. Biochem.* 16(c):142, 1992.
27. Isaacs, R. Chronic mononucleosis syndrome. *Blood* 3:858, 1948.
28. Tobi, M., Ravid, Z., Feldman-Weiss, V., et al. Prolonged atypical infection associated with serological evidence of persistent Epstein-Barr infection. *Lancet* 1:61, 1982.
29. Dubois, R. E., Seeley, J. K., Brus, I., et al. Chronic mononucleosis syndrome. *South. Med. J.* 77:1376, 1984.
30. Borysiewicz, L. K., Haworth, S. J., Cohen, J., et al. Epstein-Barr virus–specific immune defects in patients with persistent symptoms following infectious mononucleosis. *Q. J. Med.* 58:111, 1986.
31. Hotchin, N. A., Read, R., Smith, D. G., and Crawford, D. H. Active Epstein-Barr virus infection in post-viral fatigue syndrome. *J. Infect.* 18:143, 1989.
32. Archard, L. C., Peters, J. L., Behan, P. O., et al. Postviral chronic fatigue syndrome: Persistence of Epstein-Barr virus DNA in muscle. In Ablashi, D. V., et al. (eds.). *Epstein-Barr Virus and Human Disease II.* Clifton, N.J.: Humana Press, 1989. P. 439.
33. Cunningham, L., Bowles, N. E., and Archard, L. C. Persistent virus infection of muscle in postviral fatigue syndrome. *Br. Med. Bull.* 47(4):852, 1991.
34. Gow, J. W., Simpson K., Rethwilm, A., et al. Search for retrovirus in the chronic fatigue syndrome. *J. Clin. Pathol.* 45:11, 1992.
35. Koprowski, H., DeFreitas, E. C., Harper, M. E., et al. Multiple sclerosis and human T-cell lymphotropic retroviruses. *Nature* 318:154, 1985.

36. Ehrlich, G. D., Glasser, J. B., Bryz-Gornia, V., et al. Multiple sclerosis, retroviruses and PCR. *Neurology* 41:335, 1991.
37. Rozenberg, F., Lefebvre, S., Lubetzki, C., et al. Analysis of retroviral sequences in the spinal form of multiple sclerosis. *Ann. Neurol.* 29:333, 1991.
38. Southern, P., and Oldstone, M. B. A. Medical consequences of persistent viral infection. *N. Engl. J. Med.* 314:359, 1986.
39. Haywood, A. M. Patterns of persistent viral infection. *N. Engl. J. Med.* 315:939, 1986.
40. de la Torre, J. C., Borrow, P., and Oldstone, M. B. A. Viral persistence and disease: Cytopathology in the absence of cytolysis. *Br. Med. Bull.* 47(4):838, 1991.
41. Oldstone, M. B. A., Sinha, Y. N., Blount, P., et al. Virus-induced alterations in homeostasis: Alteration in differentiated functions of infected cells in vivo. *Science* 218:1125, 1982.
42. Oldstone, M. B. A., Rodriguez, M., Daughaday, W. H., and Lampert, P. W. Viral perturbation of endocrine function: Disorder of cell function leading to disturbed homeostasis and disease. *Nature* 307:278, 1984.
43. Oldstone, M. B. A. An old nemesis in new clothing: Viruses playing new tricks by causing cytopathology in the absence of cytolysis. *J. Infect. Dis.* 152:665, 1985.
44. Oldstone, M. B. A. Viral alteration of cell function. *Sci. Am.* 260:42, 1989.
45. Bocci, V. Central nervous system toxicity of interferons and other cytokines. *J. Biol. Reg. Homeo. Agents* 2(3):107, 1988.
46. Schluederberg, A., Straus, S. E., and Grufferman, S. (eds). Considerations in the design of studies of chronic fatigue syndrome. *Rev. Infect. Dis.* 13:1, 1991.
47. Frei, K., Malipero, U. V., Leist, T. P., et al. On the cellular source and function of interleukin-6 produced in the central nervous system in viral diseases. *Eur. J. Immunol.* 19:689, 1989.
48. Moskophidis, D., Frei, K., Lohler, J., et al. Production of random classes of immunoglobulins in brain tissue during persistent viral infection paralleled by secretion of interleukin-6 (IL-6) but not IL-4, IL-5 and gamma interferon. *J. Virol.* 65:1, 1991.
49. Ikemoto, N., Ronjat, M., Meszaros, L. G., and Koshita, M. Postulated role of calsequestrin in the regulation of calcium release from sarcoplasmic reticulum. *Biochem.* 28:6764, 1989.
50. Fujii, J., Willard, H., and MacLennan, D. H. Characterisation and localisation to human chromosome 1 of human fast-twitch skeletal muscle calsequestrin gene. *Som. Cell Mol. Gen.* 16:185, 1990.

Lewis Sudarsky

Central Mechanisms of Fatigue

Fatigue is a common symptom in general medicine, with many causes. In *Cecil's Textbook of Medicine* fatigue is defined as "an abnormal rate or degree of exhaustion during or following motor activity" [1]. Muscular fatigue is the cardinal symptom of myasthenia gravis, but only a small number of patients presenting with fatigue have a grave neuromuscular disease. More typically, fatigue is a nonspecific complaint expressed by patients in a primary care setting [2].

The concept of prolonged fatigue as the core feature of an infectious illness is relatively recent, following epidemics of asthenia in England, Iceland, and North America [3]. A working definition of chronic fatigue syndrome (CFS) has been assembled over the past 10 years, propelled by a renewal of interest in its cause [4,5]. The principal feature is fatigue, exacerbated by minor exercise, persisting for 6 months or longer, with 50% reduction in the patient's usual daily activity. Some patients exhibit myalgia, malaise, impaired concentration, or low-grade fever, but these features are not necessary for diagnosis. A possible diagnostic criterion is a history of an antecedent viral infection. The syndrome is broadened somewhat if the requirement for demonstrated infection is relaxed.

When considering the pathophysiology of fatigue in CFS, it is instructive to consider patients with well-defined disorders who *routinely* complain of fatigue as a disabling feature of their illness. Fatigue is a salient complaint in patients with myasthenia and in patients with metabolic disorders of skeletal muscle who have difficulty generating muscular

109

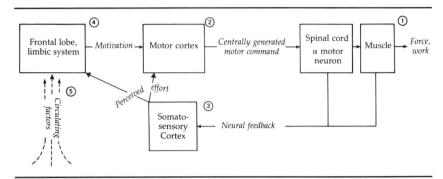

Fig. 7-1. The production of muscular effort. A simplified block diagram details the anatomy involved in muscular work. Several sites have been studied in an effort to define the mechanism for fatigue in the chronic fatigue syndrome.

work. A surprisingly large number of patients with multiple sclerosis complain of fatigue when their illness is active. The same can be said for patients with Parkinson's disease, who complain of fatigue when their medications wear off. Patients with sleep disorders typically complain of fatigue, as do patients with depression and those taking psychotropic drugs. Some viral illnesses are characterized by prominent fatigue, notably influenza, infectious mononucleosis, and AIDS. Many chronic systemic diseases produce fatigue; reduced respiratory capacity is not always at issue.

Figure 7-1 reviews the anatomy involved in the production of muscular work. Some of the possible mechanisms for fatigue in CFS are considered in this chapter. The first site (skeletal muscle and the myoneural junction) is considered in Chapter 13, and has been discussed by Edwards [8]. The focus here is on some of the upstream possibilities and the search for a central cause. Site 2 in the figure is the centrally generated motor command. A disorder here might result in inefficient utilization of muscular effort. Site 3 is the neural feedback from the musculoskeletal system, and the perceived effort (which might be out of proportion to the actual work). Site 4 places the lesion within the limbic system, resulting in a disorder of motivation—an asthenia of the will. The final mechanism to be considered is circulating factors that might influence the nervous system, resulting in a sense of exhaustion (site 5).

CENTRAL CONTROL OVER MUSCLE ACTIVATION

A variety of techniques exist for examining muscle performance with specific reference to central and peripheral correlates of fatigue. Measurement of venous lactate after exercise is sometimes used to screen for metabolic disorders of muscle, and nuclear magnetic resonance spectroscopy has been utilized to examine intracellular lactate content in muscle after exercise. A majority of CFS patients studied in this fashion have no discernible abnormality [6]. Muscle biopsy immediately after exercise has failed to show metabolic disturbance in patients with CFS [5]. Single-fiber electromyographic studies have likewise been unrevealing [7].

Physiologic measures provide indirect information about central control over motor performance, as reviewed by Edwards [8]. In a study from his laboratory in Liverpool, maximal voluntary contraction was examined in the quadriceps of 22 patients with CFS. Most patients produced normal force profiles. In the seven who generated forces below the normal range, more force could be elicited when the muscle was stimulated electrically [9]. As noted by Miller's group, chronic fatigue patients working the anterior tibial muscles at maximal voluntary contraction also demonstrate a degree of central fatigue. These patients maintained force well over a 4-minute interval, but additional reserve could be found after electrical stimulation [10].

Lloyd et al. asked 12 chronic fatigue patients to produce submaximal isometric contraction over a 45-minute endurance sequence in an attempt to reproduce in the laboratory the kind of task the patients found most fatiguing [11]. Force was comparable in patients and controls, and a 25% reduction in strength was observed over the 45 minutes for both groups. Twitch interpolation was used to examine the degree of central activation of muscle. An electrical stimulus was applied during maximum voluntary contraction to examine the reserve capacity (and the proportion of activation of muscle). The chronic fatigue patients achieved 99% maximum activation initially and 92% at the end of the endurance sequence. This activation rate was in all respects comparable to controls. While the various reports differ on this point, the data from the Lloyd study speak against a defect in central activation of muscle (site 2 in Fig. 7-1).

PERCEIVED EFFORT

Lloyd and colleagues also asked these patients to rate their degree of effort using a subjective effort scale developed by Borg et al. [12]. No significant difference in perceived exertion between patients and controls was found, though the patients rated their effort marginally higher. In this study, there was no apparent abnormality in the sensory feedback that informed the patients on muscular force levels during exercise (site 3). Lloyd concluded that "the crucial pathophysiological abnormality responsible for the prominent subjective fatigability must lie within the central nervous system above the level of the motor cortex."

MOTIVATION

The central forces that impel movement are better understood today than they were 50 years ago. The first cerebral potentials in anticipation of a voluntary movement can be recorded over central regions in the 500 msec before muscle activation. The preparation for movement involves frontal premotor areas and parallel processing circuits through the basal ganglia and cerebellum. The urge to move presumably originates elsewhere. The costs and consequences of action are pondered by the frontal lobes, which must take effort into account.

The studies of Olds and Milner on intracranial self-stimulation provide a neuroanatomic substrate for motivational aspects of behavior [13]. Stimulation of the septal area in animals, particularly along the medial forebrain bundle (the A10 dopamine pathway), seems to provide the maximal behavioral reinforcement [14]. The anterior cingulate and mesocortical dopamine systems appear to be important for motivating behavior in humans [15]. Cocaine may have some of its behavioral effect on these systems [16].

Disorders of central dopamine pathways are associated with deficits in behavioral motivation, including fatigue. Fatigue is a prominent symptom in Parkinson's disease and appears out of proportion to sedation in patients taking neuroleptic drugs. In both instances, fatigue is present prior to movement and does not strictly follow exertion. Selegeline (a monoamine oxidase B isoenzyme inhibitor) and amantadine (a dopamine releaser) have been used to treat symptoms of fatigue in multiple sclerosis as well as Parkinson's disease. The dopamine system has not been examined in CFS patients who do not otherwise appear parkinsonian.

Study of the frontal lobes and limbic system in general is a larger task. Patients often describe increased effort in mental as well as physical work. Neuropsychologic measures of performance in CFS have shown deficits in attention [17]. Hickie et al. studied 48 patients using psychiatric interview as well as psychometric testing. They found clinical evidence of depression in 46% [18]. Wessely and Powell found that 72% of patients with chronic fatigue seen at the National Hospital in London met research diagnostic criteria for a psychiatric disorder, even when fatigue was excluded as a symptom [19].

CIRCULATING FACTORS

Could the fatigue experienced by patients with CFS originate with circulating factors rather than activity in neural networks? Such a substance could be inappropriately released by skeletal muscle during exercise. Elaboration of lactate and depletion of high-energy phosphate are responsible for the pain and exhaustion normally associated with strenuous exercise and anaerobic metabolism in skeletal muscle [20]. As noted, histochemical data from muscle biopsy in CFS do not suggest a disturbance of glycolytic enzymes.

Another model for CFS is the asthenia and fatigue seen for up to 2 weeks following influenza virus infection. Symptoms are common well after the fever has passed. Fatigue may be related to activation of the immune system to clear the virus. Circulating mediators of inflammation may interact with receptors in the central nervous system, particularly in the hypothalamus where the blood-brain barrier is more permeable to large molecules. Cytokines such as interferon may be particularly active in promoting fatigue. In a study of 60 subjects receiving recombinant interferon-α for chronic hepatitis B virus infection at the Royal Free Hospital in London, fatigue and impaired concentration were common during treatment [21]; the implications for CFS were not lost on the investigators. Tumor necrosis factor and interleukin-1 reportedly have similar effects [22].

A number of immunologic abnormalities have been described in CFS, though the significance of these observations remains uncertain [2]. In one double-blind, placebo-controlled trial in which chronic fatigue patients were treated with immunoglobulin, an improvement in symptoms paralleled improvement in the patients' immune status [23]. This observation would support the hypothesis that fatigue is an expression of cross-talk between the immune system and the nervous system.

CONCLUSION

The pathogenesis of fatigue in CFS has not been established. Several lines of investigation suggest that the problem is not due to a disorder of muscle metabolism or synaptic transmission at the neuromuscular junction. Evidence is less clear with regard to central activation of skeletal muscle. Twitch interpolation studies have been interpreted as showing incomplete activation, but results may depend on motivation and the type of exertion.

The frontal lobes and limbic system need further study, particularly those areas concerned with motivation and effort. Some patients have difficulty with mental effort as well as physical work, which suggests a higher-level dysfunction (something on the left half of Figure 7-1). The relationship between CFS and depression is of particular interest, and pathophysiologic mechanisms may be common to these apparently different disorders. The role of circulating factors has recently received some attention, particularly circulating mediators of the immune response. Evidence is rather sketchy and preliminary, but the hypothesis is at least testable.

REFERENCES

1. Plum, F. Asthenia, fatigue and weakness. In Wyngaarden, J., and Smith, L. H. (eds.). *Cecil's Textbook of Medicine, 18th ed.* Philadelphia: Saunders, Pp. 2124–5.
2. Shafran, S. The chronic fatigue syndrome. *Am. J. Med.* 90:730, 1991.
3. Henderson, D. A., and Shelokov, A. Epidemic neuromyasthenia—Clinical syndrome? *N. Engl. J. Med.* 260:757, 1959.
4. Holmes, G. P., Kaplan, J. E., Gantz, N. M., et al. Chronic fatigue syndrome: A working case definition. *Ann. Intern. Med.* 108:387, 1988.
5. Behan, P. O., Behan, W. H. M., and Bell, E. J. The postviral fatigue syndrome—an analysis of the findings in 50 cases. *J. Infect.* 10:211, 1985.
6. Yonge, R. P. Magnetic resonance muscle studies: Implications for psychiatry. *J. R. Soc. Med.* 81:322, 1988.
7. Jamal, G. A., and Hansen, S. Electrophysiological studies in the postviral fatigue syndrome. *J. Neurol. Neurosurg. Psychiatry* 48:691, 1985.
8. Edwards, R. Central vs peripheral mechanisms of fatigue in exercise. *Muscle Nerve* 9 (Suppl.):39, 1986.
9. Stokes, M. J., Cooper, R. G., and Edwards, R. Normal muscle strength and fatigability in patients with effort syndromes. *Br. Med. J.* 297:1014, 1988.
10. Kent-Braun, J., Sharma, K., Chien, C., et al. Chronic fatigue syndrome: Pathophysiologic basis for muscular fatigue. *Neurology* 41 (Suppl):395, 1991.
11. Lloyd, A. R., Gandevia, S. C., and Hales, J. P. Muscle performance, voluntary activation, twitch properties and perceived effort in normal subjects and patients with the chronic fatigue syndrome. *Brain* 114:85, 1991.
12. Borg, G., Ljunggren, G., and Ceci, R. The increase of perceived exertion, aches and pain in the legs, heart rate and blood lactate during exercise on a bicycle ergometer. *Eur. J. Appl. Physiol.* 54:343, 1985.
13. Olds, J., and Milner, P. Positive reinforcement produced by electrical stimulation of septal area and other regions of rat brain. *J. Comp. Physiol. Psychol.* 47:419, 1954.
14. Routtenberg, A. The reward system of the brain. *Sci. Am.* 239:154, 1978.
15. Ross, E., and Stewart, M. Akinetic mutism from hypothalamic damage: Successful treatment with dopamine agonists. *Neurology* 31:1435, 1981.
16. Gavin, F. Cocaine addiction: Psychology and neurophysiology. *Science* 251:1580, 1991.
17. Daugherty, S., Henry, B. E., Peterson, D. L., et al. Chronic fatigue syndrome in northern Nevada. *Rev. Infect. Dis.* 13 (Suppl):39, 1991.
18. Hickie, I., Lloyd, A., Wakefield, D., and Parker, G. The psychiatric status of patients with the chronic fatigue syndrome. *Br. J. Psychiatry* 156:534, 1990.
19. Wessely, S., and Powell, R. Fatigue syndromes: A comparison of chronic "post-viral" fatigue with neuromuscular and affective disorders. *J. Neurol. Neurosurg. Psychiatry* 42:940, 1989.
20. Weiner, M. W., Moussavi, R. S., Baker, A. J. et al. Constant relationships between force, phosphate concentration, and pH in muscles with differential fatigability. *Neurology* 40:1888, 1990.
21. McDonald, E. M., Mann, A. H., Thomas, H. C. Interferons as mediators of psychiatric morbidity. *Lancet* 2:1175, 1987.
22. Moldofsky, H. Nonrestorative sleep and symptoms after a febrile illness in patients with fibrositis and chronic fatigue syndrome. *J. Rheumatol.* 16 (Suppl.):150, 1989.
23. Lloyd, A. R., Hickie, I., Wakefield, D., et al. A double-blind, placebo-controlled trial of intravenous immunoglobulin therapy in patients with chronic fatigue syndrome. *Am. J. Med.* 89:561, 1990.

8

Robert G. Miller

Neurophysiologic Assessment

Fatigue is one of the most common complaints in clinical medicine. Nonetheless, the pathophysiology of abnormal fatigue is still poorly understood in most clinical conditions characterized by excessive fatigue. It is therefore of utmost importance to define the patients' symptom of fatigue as precisely as possible. Patients with chronic fatigue syndrome (CFS) often complain of several different types of fatigue. The first is a sense of low energy that is frequently maximal upon arising in the morning with a sense of having slept poorly. A second type is characterized by abnormal mental fatigue, comparable to the exhaustion that one feels after hours of studying complicated material. A third type is fatigability in demanding physical activities that were well tolerated prior to developing symptoms. The fourth type of fatigue is a delayed recovery after fatiguing exercise. Some patients report that it may be many hours or days before they can recover back to baseline following any strenuous activity. Thus, patients have diverse definitions of fatigue, and clinicians in the past have had insufficient tools to evaluate fatigue either at the bedside or in the laboratory.

Fortunately, a number of new techniques are available that have added to our understanding of the mechanisms of fatigue, and they are discussed in this chapter. Fatigue is a complex process that is often multifactorial both in normal persons and in patients with various clinical syndromes [1–4]. To help understand fatigue in general, major mechanisms in fatigue of normal skeletal muscle will be reviewed. In CFS, the results of some neurophysiologic studies point to the presence of a form of central fatigue [5,6] (insufficient muscular activation that can be corrected by a superimposed electrical stimulus applied to the nerve or muscle) [7–9]. Most investigators have found no abnormality of nerve or muscle function [5,6,10,11]. However, some observers have reported abnormal muscle metabolism [12] and impaired excitation-contraction coupling [13]. In this chapter I will attempt to place all these findings in perspective with respect to the pathophysiology of fatigue in CFS.

MECHANISMS OF FATIGUE

Before discussing the mechanisms of fatigue in this syndrome, a brief review of the complex mechanisms of fatigue in normal individuals will be undertaken.

Impaired Activation in Muscle Fatigue

Diminished muscular force may occur as a consequence of breakdown in any of the multiple sites along the activation pathway, including the central nervous system (CNS), causing central fatigue [1], as well as failure of impulse propagation in peripheral nerve [14,15], impaired neuromuscular transmission [16,17], impaired excitation along the sarcotubular system [18–21], and altered calcium release at the level of the sarcoplasmic reticulum (excitation-contraction coupling) [22–24]. In addition, muscle fatigue may result from changes in energy metabolism and pH within the muscle cell [2,3,18,25]. Clearly, changes in energy metabolism and impairment of the contractile mechanism are important in some muscle diseases [26,27] and may be largely responsible for fatigue in normal muscle as well [2,3]. Trains of electrical stimuli have been used to study fatigue in animal [28–30] and human muscle [31–32]. These important studies have led to a classification of fatigue that depends on stimulus frequency (low-frequency and high-frequency fatigue) [22,33,34]. High-frequency fatigue appears similar to the fatigue that develops under conditions of maximum voluntary contraction, whereas low-frequency fatigue is probably comparable to that at more moderate levels of exercise. The precise physiologic correlate of these two types of electrically evoked fatigue require further investigation.

A number of studies suggest that changes in excitation-contraction coupling [22–24] or impairment of T tubule activation [35,36] may play an important role in muscle fatigue. In most studies of fatiguing exercise it has been difficult to isolate the role of excitation-contraction coupling. We have found that low-intensity exercise produces selective depression of both twitch tension and post-tetanic potentiation of the twitch with little alteration of metabolic factors within the muscle (high-energy phosphates and intracellular pH) and only minor changes in maximum voluntary contraction and evoked M waves. These findings suggest that fatigue in this setting may be almost entirely due to impaired excitation-contraction coupling.

The Metabolic Basis of Muscle Fatigue

Because exercise is associated with utilization of high-energy phosphate as well as acidification, it has been suggested that depletion of adenosine triphosphate (ATP) and phosphocreatine (PCr) [37], or accumulation of metabolites including inorganic phosphate ($H_2PO_4^-$ and HPO_4^{-2}, H^+, and adenosine diphosphate (ADP) [38], or some combination of both factors may lead to muscle fatigue [39–42].

High-Energy Phosphates

Earlier observations documented the rapid fall in PCr with little change in ATP. Thus, it was suggested that fatigue might be proportional to PCr depletion [37]. Magnetic resonance spectroscopy studies suggest that the products of high-energy phosphate hydrolysis (ADP, H^+, and $H_2PO_4^-$) may produce muscle fatigue [32,33,38–42]. Accumulation of these products may induce fatigue through kinetic mechanisms (e.g., by inhibiting the actomyosin ATPase system) [33,39]. Alternatively, fatigue may be in part produced because of diminished energy from ATP hydrolysis (ΔG ATP), i.e., by a thermodynamic mechanism.

Phosphate Accumulation

Recent evidence suggests that accumulation of metabolites within the muscle cell can directly inhibit cross-bridge formation. While ATP levels remain constant or only slightly diminished in fatigue, the products of hydrolysis—ADP, inorganic phosphates (both $H_2PO_4^-$ and HPO_4^{-2}), and H^+—all increase substantially [41,42]. The monovalent form of inorganic phosphate ($H_2PO_4^-$) seems to play a highly significant role in muscle fatigue by inhibiting cross-bridge cycling. Studies in amphibian muscle [43] and in skinned rabbit muscle fibers [44] suggest a linear relationship between the accumulation of $H_2PO_4^-$ and the declining force in muscle fatigue. Our own studies of human muscle suggest a direct relationship between $H_2PO_4^-$ and fatigue [41,42].

Role of Intracellular pH

That lactic acid accumulates in the muscle during exercise has been known for over a century [43]. However, the mechanisms by which increased acid accumulation result in muscle fatigue are not well understood. Increased H^+ could inhibit production of ATP by slowing the activity of two key enzymes, phosphorylase and phosphofructokinase [44]. In addition, the sarcoplasmic reticulum binds more calcium as pH falls [45], and therefore more calcium must be released to produce a given tension at low pH [46]. Furthermore, there is reduced sensitivity of the contractile mechanism to calcium as pH declines [46–48]. Finally, as H^+ accumulates, more monovalent phosphate is formed, which inhibits cross-bridge formation. In human quadriceps, metabolic acidosis increased susceptibility to fatigue and lowered intracellular pH in muscle biopsy tissue [49]. Further, carbon dioxide induced acidosis in mammalian muscle produced a fall of PCr [50]. Thus, it is not clear whether acidosis-induced fatigue is caused by increasing hydrogen ion or by depletion of high-energy phosphate [51,52]. Recent studies of mammalian muscle suggest that the changes in intracellular pH may not be sufficient to fully explain fatigue [53–56].

Central versus Peripheral Fatigue

Thus, fatigue may originate from several different sites in the chain of events that are required for motor control and muscle contraction. The term *central fatigue* refers to impaired activation of muscle on the basis of a breakdown primarily within the CNS. Potential causes of central fatigue include abnormal activation of corticospinal motor neurons as a result of a number of different pathologic processes including cell death (e.g., infarction, tumor, etc.) or demyelination (e.g., multiple sclerosis), or from limited effort in muscle activation as a result of pain, reduced motivation, limited concentration, and similar factors. Thus, failure to recruit motor neurons or to mount high discharge frequencies during muscle contraction is usually a result of central fatigue.

The standard technique for evaluating whether fatigue is central or peripheral is to superimpose a maximal electrical stimulus on the motor nerve innervating the muscle under study [7,8]. During maximal muscular activation, a superimposed electrical stimulus (either single or in a train) will elicit no additional force generation. If the muscle is incompletely activated as a result of either reduced recruitment or inadequate discharge frequencies, then additional force will be recorded in response to the superimposed electrical stimulus. When there is evidence of fatigue (defined here as declining force generation during repeated or sustained muscle contraction), and no additional force is generated in response to electrical stimulation, then the fatigue can be considered peripheral.

Peripheral fatigue may result from a defect beyond the site of stimulation of the motor nerve [57]. This could include abnormalities in the function of peripheral nerve, neuromuscular junction, excitation-contraction coupling (muscle membrane excitability, transverse tubule, calcium release from the sarcoplasmic reticulum), or cross-bridge cycling.

Fatigue in normal muscle depends on the type of exercise, the subject's degree of training, and the fiber type composition of the muscle involved. In highly motivated subjects, central fatigue is usually a minor factor. Some muscles are more difficult than others to activate in a continuous fashion, however. Both the diaphragm and the gastrocnemius are extremely difficult to fully activate, even briefly [58]. Thus, central fatigue does depend on the muscle in question, but most limb muscles can be fully activated by motivated normal subjects and central fatigue plays a relatively small role in the declining force generation. High-intensity exercise produces metabolic changes within muscle, as reviewed above, that play a major role in muscle fatigue [2,3]. Low-intensity exercise, on the other hand, appears to produce fatigue primarily through altered excitation-contraction coupling [4,22]. Recovery rates also differ, depending on the type of exercise and its duration. Metabolic changes tend to recover rapidly, usually within 15 minutes [56], while excitation-contraction coupling may take many hours to completely recover [4,22].

TECHNIQUES FOR ANALYZING FATIGUE

Needle electromyography (EMG) and nerve conduction studies are widely used to evaluate diseases affecting the nerve and muscle. Nerve conduction studies demonstrate abnormal impulse transmission or reduced evoked muscle action potentials in neurogenic disorders. With needle EMG, abnormal spontaneous activity yields objective evidence of interrupted innervation of muscle fibers, and abnormal configuration of motor unit potentials provides information about structural changes occurring within the motor unit [59]. Quantitative studies of the duration, amplitude, and polyphasic wave activity of motor unit potentials are sensitive methods for analyzing the configuration of motor unit potentials in disorders of the peripheral nerve or in myopathies [60]. Impaired motor unit recruitment can also be evaluated using needle EMG. In patients with central disorders of motor control, motor units are not fully recruited and discharge frequencies remain low or synchronization may be observed. In myopathies, the amplitude and duration of motor unit potentials are reduced and recruitment of motor units is early and full, even in weak muscles. In peripheral nerve disorders, motor unit potentials are enlarged and recruitment patterns are reduced, reflecting a decrease in the size of the motor unit pool. Routine electroencephalography can be useful in detecting areas of focal brain dysfunction that may account for impaired motor control. Generalized slowing of brain wave activity can also be detected that correlates with impaired concentration and cognitive function. These tests are relatively inexpensive and widely available. EMG and nerve conduction studies are mainly useful in ruling out neuromuscular diseases presenting with fatigue, such as myasthenia gravis.

Single-Fiber EMG

Neuromuscular transmission may be evaluated with repetitive nerve stimulation, a test that is particularly useful in clinical disorders of the neuromuscular junction such as myasthenia gravis or the Lambert-Eaton myasthenic syndrome. Single-fiber EMG is a more sensitive method of detecting abnormal neuromuscular transmission [61]. The technique allows quantitative comparison of the discharge pattern of two individual muscle fibers innervated by the same peripheral nerve. The variable interval between the discharge of the two fibers, referred to as jitter, is small in normal subjects. The variability is accounted for by different times for impulse propagation along intramuscular nerve twigs, across the neuromuscular junction, and along individual muscle fiber membranes. Abnormal jitter (mean value, < 55 μsec) reflects an abnormality of neuromuscular transmission. Clinical fatigue, such as that seen in myasthenia gravis, is virtually always associated with a second major finding on single-fiber EMG studies, termed *blocking* [61,62]. The failure of one of the pairs of muscle fibers under analysis to depolarize constitutes blocking, which is an important sign of abnormal neuromuscular transmission. Single-fiber EMG requires an expert with extensive training and is available in only a limited number of major medical centers.

Evoked Potentials

A number of techniques have been developed to evaluate impulse propagation within the CNS. Electrical stimulation of motor nerves produces somatosensory evoked potentials that can be recorded on the scalp overlying the sensory cortex of the brain. These pathways primarily involve the dorsal columns but are also abnormal in patients with corticospinal tract abnormalities. Motor control pathways may be more directly evaluated by either electrical or magnetic stimulation of the cortex of the brain [63]. Specialized electrical stimulators that generate extremely high intensity pulses of very brief duration are in use in a few centers to stimulate central motor pathways and record evoked potentials in limb muscles. Magnetic stimulators are also available that have the great advantage of being painless. Stimulation, either electrical or magnetic, may be delivered to the cortex or to the cervical spinal cord to evaluate central motor conduction.

Evoked potentials may also be used to study cognitive processes in patients with disorders of motor control and fatigue [64]. Multimodality sensory evoked potentials and auditory event-related cognitive potentials appear to result from synchronous neural activity following a particular process or stimulus. A characteristic response has been identified following a particular stimulus or event with a latency of approximately 300 msec, and has come to be known as the P300. The latency varies with the complexity of the task. Such cognitive potentials seem to relate to specific cognitive processes including memory, attention, and the evaluation of different stimuli [64]. These cognitive potentials and the evaluation of central motor conduction pathways are available only at large, specialized medical centers.

Nuclear Magnetic Resonance Spectroscopy

Magnetic resonance spectroscopy is a new technique that permits the continuous analysis of muscle metabolism in a noninvasive manner to help clarify mechanisms of fatigue in normal muscle and in patients with complaints of excessive fatigability [26]. During exercise, PCr, inorganic phosphate, intracellular pH, ATP, and lactate levels can be continuously monitored. In patients with mitochondrial myopathy, there is an elevated ratio of inorganic phosphate to PCr in resting muscle and delayed resynthesis of PCr during recovery after exercise [27]. In patients with defective glycolysis or glycogenolysis, no intracellular acidification occurs during exercise [65]. Thus, abnormal muscle metabolism may be detected with no risk or harm to the patient during fatiguing exercise. At this time, only a few specialized medical centers have this capability.

Studies of Strength, Muscle Endurance, and Excitation-Contraction Coupling

Of course, the most important property of skeletal muscle is to generate force. We define fatigue as the reduction in force generation during repeated or sustained muscle contraction [1]. Although this seems redundant, it is worth reiterating since none of the techniques already mentioned deal with the measurement of force generation per se. Thus, it is critically important when investigating fatigue to measure the changes in force generation of the exercising muscle and to correlate them with the mechanical and electrical responses to electrical stimulation, both during fatiguing exercise and during recovery.

Standardized muscle exercise protocols have been developed in our laboratory over the past 10 years [4,9,41,42,56,66]. A 4-minute sustained maximum voluntary contraction is a high-intensity exercise and produces substantial muscle fatigue that appears to depend primarily upon metabolic changes in muscle [41,42,46]. Nonetheless, other contributing factors in fatigue can be evaluated during such a protocol. The added force in response to superimposed electrical stimulation defines the amount of central fatigue, as discussed. The change in shape and area of the evoked compound muscle action potential in response to electrical stimulation provides insight into the presence of neuromuscular transmission failure or abnormal muscle membrane excitation and impulse propagation [4,67]. A change in the twitch tension, when compared with changes in the evoked compound muscle action potential, permits evaluation of excitation-contraction coupling [4,22]. Each of these measures is also utilized in a low-intensity exercise protocol that involves 6 seconds of contraction and 4 seconds of rest, initially at 30% of the maximum voluntary contraction strength for 15 minutes, and then at 50% of the maximum voluntary contraction strength for 10 minutes [4]. This protocol produces primarily a nonmetabolic fatigue that depends on impaired excitation-contraction coupling. These methods yield quantitative data about muscle fatigue and provide some insight into the mechanisms of fatigue in individual patients.

FINDINGS IN PATIENTS WITH CFS

Standard Clinical Neurophysiology

Motor and sensory nerve conduction studies have been completely normal in patients with CFS [68]. Similarly, needle EMG studies have disclosed no significant spontaneous activity and no change in the configuration of motor unit potentials. Grouped motor unit potential discharges at low frequencies have been described in some patients with CFS [68]. Simultaneous activation of agonist and antagonist muscles has been observed, suggesting a functional component to the complaint of weakness. The presence of low firing rates when maximum patient effort is requested reflects a pattern that is often seen with submaximal effort. Electroencephalography is usually normal in CFS patients in our experience.

Single-Fiber EMG

In one study, abnormal jitter was found in 75% of 40 patients with CFS [13]. However, impulse blocking was not observed even though very high values of jitter (up to 500 μsec) were recorded in some patients. In other studies of CFS, increased jitter without impulse blocking has been observed but in a much smaller proportion of patients (4 of 30 cases) [69]. The abnormal jitter has been ascribed to disuse [5], but its cause remains unclear. Certainly increased jitter is of diagnostic importance in myasthenia gravis, but it is the presence of impulse blocking that correlates with clinical evidence of fatigue [61,62]. The absence of blocking in these patients suggests that the increased jitter is a nonspecific finding with uncertain clinical significance [5,11].

Evoked Potential Studies

Standard visual, auditory, and somatosensory evoked potential studies have been entirely normal in patients with CFS [64]. However, latencies of the cognitive evoked potentials were prolonged, particularly for the P300 response. Also, reaction times from the onset of a tone to the pressing of a button were significantly prolonged in CFS patients compared with controls [64]. These results were interpreted as indicating deficits in attention and slower information processing. The authors pointed out that similar findings have not been observed in patients with depression [70].

Both magnetic stimulation applied to the scalp and electrical stimulation of the cervical spinal cord were utilized to evoke responses from an intrinsic hand muscle to evaluate central motor conduction in 9 patients with CFS [71]. Patients were studied both before and after fatiguing exercise using both types of stimulation. In all patients, central motor conduction times were normal and amplitudes of the evoked responses were preserved with no decline following fatiguing exercise [71]. These findings constitute strong evidence that impulse propagation is normal in the motor pathways of patients with CFS. Moreover, there is no evidence for reduced impulse propagation in central motor pathways as a result of fatiguing exercise.

Nuclear Magnetic Resonance Spectroscopy

In a single well-studied patient with CFS, early intramuscular acidification was demonstrated in response to fatiguing exercise [12]. The authors interpreted this finding as indicative of excessive lactic acid formation arising from a disorder of muscle metabolic regulation. The index case did have a predominance of type 2 muscle fibers on muscle biopsy, which may have contributed to the excessive fatigability and early intracellular acidification. Other investigators have disputed the clinical significance of this finding, and suggested that premature acidosis is unusual [72,73].

In order to examine the issue further, both high-intensity and low-intensity exercise of the tibialis anterior muscle was undertaken by seven patients with CFS and by sedentary, age-matched control subjects [6]. There were no significant differences in muscle fatigability in either exercise protocol, nor in patterns of recovery, in CFS patients compared with controls. There was actually slightly less acidification and a somewhat smaller accumulation of inorganic phosphate in the patients compared with controls, but the differences were not significant. Of particular interest was the finding of substantial added force in response to superimposed electrical stimulation during the sustained exercise protocol. Thus, these results fail to provide support for any disorder of muscle metabolism in patients with CFS but do indicate a significant component of central fatigue based on the substantial added force.

Strength, Endurance, and Excitation-Contraction Coupling

Normal strength and endurance of intermittent maximum voluntary contraction of the elbow flexors in 20 patients with CFS were reported in one recent investigation [11]. In another study of 30 patients with the disorder, studies were carried out on the quadriceps muscle as well as the abductor pollicis and cycle ergometry was performed to the point of exhaustion [5]. The studies on the abductor pollicis depended only on electrical stimulation in order to remove all voluntary influence on the evaluation of muscular endurance. There were no significant differences between force generation or fatigability of patients compared with controls in the electrically stimulated fatiguing exercise. The maximum voluntary contraction strength of the quadriceps was reduced in some patients but added force was observed in response to superimposed electrical stimulation, indicating incomplete muscular activation. Cycle ergometry produced slightly lower maximum heart rates, indicating lower effort in the patients with CFS. The authors concluded that there must be increased central fatigue rather than any peripheral fatigue in these patients [5]. Others have found normal aerobic work capacity in CFS patients [74]. Our own studies of patients with CFS also suggest a substantial component of central fatigue, as mentioned earlier [6].

A follow-up study from the same laboratory demonstrated two important findings [75]. First, patients with CFS had a higher rating of perceived effort in fatiguing exercise compared with controls for the same degree of increased heart rate during bicycle exercise. Second, the rate of recovery after fatiguing exercise was similar in patients and in controls. Thus, both exercise performance and recovery were essentially normal in CFS patients, but perceived fatigue was more pronounced for a given workload.

Other studies have been designed to examine excitation-contraction coupling and muscle membrane function in CFS patients [6,10]. Compound muscle action potential amplitudes were preserved in patients and in controls immediately after a 4-minute sustained maximum voluntary contraction [6]. This observation suggests that propagation of impulses along the muscle membrane is normal in patients with CFS, so at least this portion of excitation-contraction coupling is normal. In general, the process of excitation-contraction coupling is difficult to evaluate in human muscle. Recent evidence suggests that either reduced calcium release from the sarcoplasmic reticulum or abnormal impulse propagation in the transverse tubule may play a major role in some types of fatigue of human muscle, but neither can be evaluated in human muscle at this time [35,36,76].

An exercise protocol was specifically designed to simulate everyday activity and evaluate excitation-contraction coupling in the elbow flexor muscles of patients with CFS [10]. Twelve patients and controls carried out intermittent low-intensity exercise (30% maximum voluntary contraction, 6 seconds contraction, 4 seconds rest) for 45 minutes with a sustained maximum voluntary contraction of 3 seconds every 5 minutes to evaluate fatigue. Both a subjective rating of perceived effort and superimposed electrical stimulation to evaluate central fatigue were utilized in this study. No difference in fatigue, voluntary force generation, central fatigue, or perceived effort was found between the two groups. Thus, no abnormality of excitation-contraction coupling could be identified in patients with CFS [10]. The findings in our own laboratory, with a somewhat different protocol, also revealed no abnormality of excitation-contraction coupling [6].

CONCLUSION

Thus, no evidence of peripheral fatigue or of any clinically significant abnormality of nerve or muscle function has been found in patients with CFS. It is true that patients with mitochondrial myopathies and other neuromuscular diseases may be misdiagnosed as having CFS, but this is rare [77,78]. The absence of a metabolic disorder in recent studies of CFS patients is consistent with the lack of significant abnormalities on both light and electron microscopic examination of muscle biopsies as well as the normal findings in biochemical analysis of glycolytic and mitochondrial enzymes in muscle tissue [79].

In high-intensity exercise, however, there is evidence that impaired muscle activation and central fatigue do contribute to muscle fatigue in CFS [5,6]. The finding of increasing central fatigue during demanding exercise protocols is consistent with reports of abnormal cognitive potentials that point to problems with concentration and attention in CFS patients [64]. The functional integrity of the central motor pathways appears to be preserved based on both electrical and magnetic stimulation of these pathways before and after exercise [71]. Other factors in central fatigue have not been subjected to systematic study in CFS. For example, during prolonged exhausting exercise, branched-chain amino acids are reduced in the serum of normal subjects, which may alter the perception of fatigue through changes in neurotransmitter levels in the brain [80]. Also, afferent feedback from small somatic nerve endings in fatigued muscle may be important in the perception of fatigue, which seems to be exaggerated in chronic fatigue patients [81]. At this time, most of the available evidence suggests that the major source of fatigue in patients with CFS resides outside of the motor control system [82]. However, the precise interaction between physiologic and psychologic alterations that contribute to the increased perception of fatigue remains unclear. Further studies of factors that contribute to central fatigue may be fruitful.

REFERENCES

1. Edwards, R. H. T. Human muscle function and fatigue. In R. Porter and J. Whelan (eds.). *Human Muscle Fatigue: Physiological Mechanisms* (Ciba Foundation Symposium 82). London: Pitman Medical, 1981. Pp. 1–18.
2. Baker, A. J., Carson, P. J., Miller, R. G., and Weiner, M. W. Investigations of muscle bioenergetics with ^{31}P NMR. *Invest. Radiol.* 24:1001, 1989.
3. Weiner, M. W., Baker, A., Carson, P., et al. Noninvasive techniques in

biology and medicine. In S. E. Freeman, E. Fukushima, and E. R. Greene (eds.). *³¹P MRS Studies of Skeletal Muscle and Heart: Evidence of Metabolic Regulation by Inorganic Phosphate.* San Francisco: San Francisco Press, 1990. Pp. 111–122.

4. Moussavi, R. S., Carson, P. J., Boska, M. D., et al. Nonmetabolic fatigue in exercising human muscle. *Neurology* 39:1222, 1989.

5. Stokes, M. J., Cooper, R. G., and Edwards, R. H. T. Normal muscle strength and fatigability in patients with effort syndromes. *Br. Med. J.* 297:1014, 1988.

6. Kent-Braun, J., Sharma, K., Chien, C., et al. Chronic fatigue syndrome: Pathophysiologic basis for muscular fatigue. *Neurology* 41(Suppl.):395, 1991.

7. Belanger, A. Y., and McComas, A. J. Extent of motor unit activation during effort. *J. Appl. Physiol.* 51:1131, 1981.

8. Bigland-Ritchie, B., Burbush, F., and Woods, J. J. Fatigue of intermittent submaximal voluntary contractions: Central and peripheral factors. *J. Appl. Physiol.* 61:421, 1986.

9. Milner-Brown, H. S., Mellenthin, M., and Miller, R. G. Quantifying human muscle strength, endurance and fatigue. *Arch. Phys. Med. Rehabil.* 67:530, 1986.

10. Lloyd, A. R., Hales, J. P., and Gandevia, S. C. Muscle strength, endurance and recovery in the post-infection fatigue syndrome. *J. Neurol. Neurosurg. Psychiatry* 51:1316, 1988.

11. Lloyd, R., Gandevia, S. C., and Hales, J. P. Muscle performance, voluntary activation, twitch properties and perceived effort in normal subjects and patients with the chronic fatigue syndrome. *Brain* 114:85, 1991.

12. Arnold, D. L., Bore, P. J., Radda, G. K., et al. Excessive intracellular acidosis of skeletal muscle on exercise in a patient with a post-viral exhaustion/fatigue syndrome—A ³¹P nuclear magnetic resonance study. *Lancet* 1:1367, 1984.

13. Jamal, G. A., and Hansen, S. Electrophysiological studies in the post-viral fatigue syndrome. *J. Neurol. Neurosurg. Psychiatry* 48:691, 1985.

14. Smith, D. O. Mechanisms of action potential propagation failure at sites of axon branching in the crayfish. *J. Physiol.* 301:243, 1980.

15. Swadlow, H. A., Kocsis, D., and Waxman, S. G. Modulation of impulse conduction along the axonal tree. *Annu. Rev. Biophys. Bioeng.* 9:143, 1980.

16. Kugelberg, E., and Lindegren, B. Transmission and contraction fatigue of rat motor units in relation to succinate dehydrogenase activity of motor unit fibers. *J. Physiol.* 288:285, 1979.

17. Krnjevic, K., and Miledi, R. Failure of neuromuscular propagation in rats. *J. Physiol.* 140:440, 1958.

18. Merton, P. A. Voluntary strength and fatigue. *J. Physiol.* 128:553, 1954.

19. Stephens, J. A., and Taylor, A. Fatigue of maintained voluntary muscle contraction in man. *J. Physiol.* 220:1, 1972.

20. Bigland-Ritchie, B., Kukulka, C. G., Lippold, O. C. J., and Woods, J. J. The absence of neuromuscular transmission failure in sustained maximal voluntary contractions. *J. Physiol.* 330:265, 1982.

21. Milner-Brown, H.S., and Miller, R. G. Muscle membrane excitation and impulse propagation velocity are reduced during muscle fatigue. *Muscle Nerve* 9:367, 1986.

22. Edwards, R. H. T., Hill, D. K., Jones, D. A., and Merton, P. A. Fatigue of long duration in human skeletal muscle after exercise. *J. Physiol.* 272:769, 1977.

23. Eberstein, A., and Sandow, A. Fatigue mechanisms in muscle fibres. In *The Effect of Use and Disuse on Neuromuscular Function.* Prague: National Academy of Czechoslovakia, 1963. Pp. 515–526.

24. Nassar-Gentina, V., Passonneau, J. V., and Rapoport, S. I. Fatigue and

metabolism in frog muscle fibers during stimulation and in response to caffeine. *Am. J. Physiol.* 241:C160, 1981.

25. Wilkie, D. R. Shortage of chemical fuel as a cause of fatigue: Studies by nuclear magnetic resonance and bicycle ergometry. In R. Porter and J. Whelan (eds.). *Human Muscle Fatigue: Physiological Mechanisms* (Ciba Foundation Symposium 82). London: Pitman Medical, 1981. Pp. 102–119.

26. Miller, R. G., Carson, P. J., Moussavi, R. S., et al. The use of magnetic resonance spectroscopy to evaluate muscular fatigue and human muscle disease. *Appl. Radiol.* 18:33, 1989.

27. Argov, Z., and Bank, W. Phosphorus magnetic resonance spectroscopy (^{31}P MRS) in neuromuscular disorders. *Ann. Neurol.* 30:90, 1991.

28. Clamann, H. P., and Robinson, A. J. A comparison of electromyographic and mechanical fatigue properties in motor units of the cat hindlimb. *Brain Res.* 327:203, 1985.

29. Burke, R. E. Motor units: Anatomy, physiology, and functional organization. In J. M. Brookhart and V. B. Mountcastle (eds.). *Handbook of Physiology, Section J, Neurophysiology, Vol II, Part I: Motor Control.* Baltimore: Williams & Wilkins, 1981.

30. Stuart, D. G., and Enoka, R. M. Motoneurons, motor units, and the size principle. In R. N. Rosenberg and W. D. Willis (eds.). *The Clinical Neurosciences, Section 5, Chapter 17, Neurobiology.* New York: Churchill Livingstone, 1983.

31. Edwards, R. H. T., and Wiles, C. M. Energy exchange in human skeletal muscle during isometric contraction. *Circ. Res.* 48(Suppl 1):11, 1981.

32. Edwards, R. H. T. Weakness and fatigue of skeletal muscles. *Adv. Med.* 18:100, 1982.

33. Bigland-Ritchie, B. EMG/force relations and fatigue of human voluntary contractions. In D. I. Miller (ed). *Exercise and Sports Sciences Reviews* (American College of Sports Medicine Series), 1981.

34. Bigland-Ritchie, B., Jones, D. A., and Woods, J. J. Excitation frequency and muscle fatigue: Electrical responses during human voluntary and stimulated contractions. *Exp. Neurol.* 64:414, 1979.

35. Lannergren, J., and Westerblad, H. Force and membrane potential during and after fatiguing, continuous high-frequency stimulation of single *Xenopus* muscle fibres. *Acta Physiol. Scand.* 128:359, 1986.

36. Lannergren, J., and Westerblad, H. Action potential fatigue in single skeletal muscle fibres of *Xenopus. Acta Physiol. Scand.* 129:311, 1987.

37. Spande, J. I., and Schottelius, B. A. Chemical basis of fatigue in isolated mouse soleus muscle. *Am. J. Physiol.* 219:1490, 1970.

38. Dawson, M. J., Gadian, D. G., and Wilkie, D. R. Contraction and recovery of living muscle studied by ^{31}P nuclear magnetic resonance. *J. Physiol.* 267:703, 1977.

39. Wilkie, D. R. Muscular fatigue: Effects of hydrogen ions and inorganic phosphate. *Fed. Proc.* 45:2921, 1986.

40. Radda, G. K. The use of NMR spectroscopy for the understanding of disease. *Science* 233:640, 1986.

41. Miller, R. G., Boska, M. D., Moussavi, M. S., et al. ^{31}NMR studies of high-energy phosphates and pH in human muscle fatigue: Comparison of aerobic and anaerobic exercise. *J. Clin. Invest.* 81:1190, 1988.

42. Weiner, M. W., Moussavi, R. S., Baker, A. J., et al. Constant relationships between force, phosphate concentration, and pH in muscles with differential fatigability. *Neurology* 40:1888, 1990.

43. Lehman, C. F. *Lehrbuch der physiologischen Chemie,* 1850.

44. Hermansen, L. Effect of metabolic changes on force generations in skeletal

muscle during maximal exercise. In R. Porter and J. Whelan (eds.). *Human Muscle Fatigue: Physiological Mechanisms* (Ciba Foundation Symposium 82). London: Pitman Medical, 1981.

45. Nakamura, Y., and Schwartz, A. Possible control of intracellular calcium metabolism by [H$^+$]: Sarcoplasmic reticulum of skeletal and cardiac muscle. *Biochem. Biophys. Res. Commun.* 41:830, 1970.

46. Robertson, S., and Kerrick, W. The effect of pH on submaximal and maximal Ca^{2+}-activated tension in skinned frog skeletal fibers. *Biophys. J.* 16:73A(abstr.), 1976.

47. Schadler, M. Proportionale Aktivierung von ATP-ase-Aktivität und Kontraktionsspannung durch Calciumionen in isolierten kontraktilen Strukturen verschiedenen Muskelarten. *Pfluegers Arch. Ges. Physiol.* 296:70, 1967.

48. Donaldson, S. K., Hermansen, L., and Bolles, L. Differential, direct effect of H$^+$ on Ca^{2+}-activated force of skinned fibers from the soleus, cardiac and adductor magnus muscles of rabbits. *Pfluegers Arch. Eur. J. Physiol.* 376:55, 1978.

49. Hultman, E., Del Canale, S., and Sjoholm, H. Effect of induced metabolic acidosis on intracellular pH, buffer capacity and contraction force of human skeletal muscle. *Clin. Sci.* 69:505, 1985.

50. Sahlin, K., Edström, L., Sjöholm, H., et al. Effects of lactic acid accumulation and ATP decrease in muscle tension and relaxation. *Am. J. Physiol.* 240:121, 1981.

51. Sahlin, K., Edstron, L., and Sjoholm, N. Fatigue and phosphocreatine depletion during carbon dioxide–induced acidosis in rat muscle. *Am. J. Physiol.* 245:C15, 1983.

52. Sahlin, K. Intracellular pH and energy metabolism in skeletal muscle of man. *Acta Physiol. Scand. [Suppl.]* 455:2, 1978.

53. Benaud, J. M., Allard, J., and Mainwood, G. W. Is the change in intracellular pH during fatigue large enough to be the main cause of fatigue? *Can. J. Physiol. Pharmacol.* 64:764, 1986.

54. Renaud, J. M., and Mainwood, G. W. The interactive effects of fatigue and pH on the ionic conductance of frog sartorius muscle fiber. *Can. J. Physiol. Pharmacol.* 63:1444, 1985.

55. Renaud, J. M., and Mainwood, G. W. The effects of pH on the kinetics of fatigue and recovery in frog sartorius muscle. *Can. J. Physiol. Pharmacol.* 63:1435, 1985.

56. Boska, M. D., Moussavi, R. S., Carson, P. J., et al. The metabolic basis of recovery after fatiguing exercise of human muscle. *Neurology* 40:240, 1990.

57. Jones, D. A. Muscle fatigue due to changes beyond the neuromuscular junction. In R. Porter and J. Whelan (eds.). *Muscle Fatigue: Physiological Mechanisms* (Ciba Foundation Symposium 82). London: Pitman Medical, 1981. Pp. 178–196.

58. Belanger, A. Y., and McComas, A. J. Extent of motor unit activation during effort. *J. Appl. Physiol.* 51:1131, 1981.

59. Daube, J. R. Needle examination in clinical electromyography. *Muscle Nerve* 14:685, 1991.

60. Buchthal, F., and Kamieniecka, Z. The diagnostic yield of quantified electromyography and quantified muscle biopsy in neuromuscular disorders. *Muscle Nerve* 5:265, 1982.

61. Keesey, J. C. Electrodiagnostic approach to defects of neuromuscular transmission. *Muscle Nerve* 12:613, 1989.

62. Sanders, D. G., and Howard, J. F., Jr. Single-fiber electromyography in myasthenia gravis. *Muscle Nerve* 9:809, 1986.

63. Eisen, A. A., and Shtybel, W. Clinical experience with transcranial magnetic stimulation. *Muscle Nerve* 13:995, 1990.

64. Prasher, D., Smith, A., and Findley, L. Sensory and cognitive event-related potentials in myalgic encephalomyelitis. *J. Neurol. Neurosurg. Psychiatry* 53:247, 1990.

65. Ross, B. D., Radda, G. K., Gadian, D. G., et al. Examination of a case of suspected McArdle's syndrome by nuclear magnetic resonance. *N. Engl. J. Med.* 304:1338, 1981.

66. Miller, R. G., Giannini, D., and Milner-Brown, H. S. Effects of fatiguing exercise on high-energy phosphates, force, and EMG: Evidence for three phases of recovery. *Muscle Nerve* 10:810, 1987.

67. Milner-Brown, H. S., and Miller, R. G. Muscle membrane excitation and impulse propagation velocity are reduced during muscle fatigue. *Muscle Nerve* 9:367, 1986.

68. Thomas, P. K. Postviral fatigue syndrome. *Lancet* 2:218, 1987.

69. Roberts, L. J. Single fiber EMG studies in the chronic fatigue syndrome. *J. Neurol. Sci.* 98 (Suppl):97, 1990.

70. Patterson, J. V., Michalewski, H. J., and Starr, A. Latency variability of the components of auditory event-related potentials to infrequent stimuli in aging, Alzheimer-type dementia and depression. *Electroencephalogr. Clin. Neurophysiol.* 71:450, 1988.

71. Waddy, H., Wessely, S., and Murray, N. M. F. Central motor conduction studies in chronic-postviral fatigue syndrome. *Electroencephalogr. Clin. Neurophysiol.* 75(Suppl.):S160, 1990.

72. Wagenmakers, A., Coakley, J., and Edwards, R. H. T. The metabolic consequences of reduced habitual activities in patients with muscle pain and disease. *Ergonomics* 31:1519, 1988.

73. Lewis, S., and Haller, R. Physiologic measurement of exercise and fatigue with special reference to chronic fatigue syndrome. *Rev. Infect. Dis.* 13 (Suppl. 1):98, 1991.

74. Riley, M., O'Brien, C., McCluskey, D., et al. Aerobic work capacity in patients with chronic fatigue syndrome. *Br. Med. J.* 301:953, 1990.

75. Gibson, H., Carroll, N., Coakley, J., and Edwards, R. H. T. Recovery from maximal exercise in chronic fatigue states. *J.Neurol. Sci.* 98 (Suppl.):97, 1990.

76. Allen, D. G., Lee, J. A., and Westerblad, H. Intracellular calcium and tension during fatigue in isolated single muscle fibres from *Xenopus laevis*. *J. Physiol.* 415:433, 1989.

77. Karpati, G., Carpenter, S., Weller, B., and Massa, R. Muscle biopsy experience in the chronic fatigue syndrome. *J. Neurol. Sci.* 98 (Suppl.):96, 1990.

78. Pelekanos, J. T., Brooke, M. H., Hanstock, C., et al. Cytochrome oxidase deficiency presenting as a fatigue syndrome. *Neurology* 40 (Suppl. 1):122, 1990.

79. Shafran, S. D. The chronic fatigue syndrome. *Am. J. Med.* 90:730, 1991.

80. Blomstrand, E., Celsing, F., Newsholme, E. A., et al. Changes in plasma concentration of aromatic and branched-chain amino acids during sustained exercise in man and their possible role in fatigue. *Acta Physiol. Scand.* 133:115, 1988.

81. Woods, J. J., Furbush, F. Bigland-Ritchie, B., et al. Evidence for a fatigue-induced reflex inhibition of motoneuron firing rates. *J. Physiol.* 58:125, 1987.

82. Wessely, S. Chronic fatigue syndrome. *J. Neurol. Neurosurg. Psychiatry* 54:669, 1991.

9

Wilhelmina M. H. Behan
Ian Downie
Ian A. R. More
Peter O. Behan

Changes in Muscle Mitochondria

Epidemics of a curious neuromuscular disease were first reported from America in the 1930s but have now been recognized worldwide. A plethora of names has been given to the illness, many indicating the geographic location (e.g., Akureyri or Iceland disease, Royal Free disease), others concentrating on one or more of the varied and apparently vague symptoms, for example, atypical poliomyelitis or benign diencephalitis (reviewed in [1]). After the biggest epidemic in Britain—the outbreak at the Royal Free Hospital—an astute general practitioner in the region, Dr. A. M. Ramsay, pointed out that he had seen several sporadic cases before the epidemic started, and was now again seeing single affected patients [2]. He concluded that the disorder was an epidemic disease with an endemic prevalence in the community. It is plain that the endemic cases are the ones which are more commonly seen at present [1,3].

The main presenting symptom in all patients is fatigue, with or without myalgia. This is reflected in the two names now used: the postviral fatigue syndrome (PFS) for cases developing after an acute viral type of illness [1], and the chronic fatigue syndrome (CFS) when the onset is insidious [4]. Central nervous system manifestations, including disturbance of sleep and appetite, loss of concentration, and subtle immunologic deficits, are also part of the picture [1,4].

It has previously been difficult to make a definite diagnosis in these patients because their principal symptom, fatigue, is such an ill-defined subjective sensation. Now that diagnostic guidelines [5] and a working case definition [4] have been laid down, cases should be identified more easily. It must be recognized, however, that because clinical signs of neuromuscular disease are rarely detectable and routine laboratory evidence of muscle breakdown is seldom found, there is a tendency to categorize the syndrome as a psychiatric disorder [6], at which point scientific investigations seem to cease abruptly.

The results of highly specialized tests show undeniable evidence of muscle dysfunction in these patients. Single-fiber electromyography suggests a defect in the muscle fiber membrane [7]. On ^{31}P nuclear magnetic resonance testing, the pattern of inorganic phosphate, phosphocreatine, and adenosine triphosphate (ATP) concentrations after exercise shows abnormalities in keeping with the unusually early onset of fatigue and suggestive of interference in the coordination of oxidative and anaerobic metabolism [8,9]. It was therefore of great interest when we identified morphologic mitochondrial abnormalities in the muscle biopsies of patients with CFS. We reported the findings in a preliminary study [10].

Since then, muscle biopsies of 150 very well-characterized patients with the postviral fatigue syndrome (PFS) from the Institute of Neurological Sciences in Glasgow have been studied. The results were compared to the following subject groups: (1) a surgical control group consisting of 50 patients of the same age and sex, with no muscle diseases, admitted for routine surgical procedures and from whom 1 mm^3 specimens could be taken at operation; (2) 50 patients with mixed connective tissue diseases, including polymyositis; and (3) five patients with mitochondrial myopathies.

The muscle biopsy specimens consisted of two cores of skeletal muscle from the right vastus lateralis, taken with the UCH biopsy needle under local anesthesia as previously described [11]. The tissue received was divided into three parts: two small (1 mm^3) fragments for electron microscopy and viral nucleic acid analysis respectively, and the remainder for histologic, histochemical, and in situ molecular hybridization studies. The specimens were frozen or fixed in glutaraldehyde and processed as described [11]. The mitochondria were then examined morphologically and measured using an image analyzer.

MORPHOLOGIC ABNORMALITIES IN CFS

Light microscopic examination added very little to what has already been reported [1,3]: the most common finding on the frozen sections in both male and female patients was atrophy of type 2 fibers, ranging from mild and focal to moderately severe and diffuse. This nonspecific finding, present in many systemic illnesses and also associated with disuse [12], is obviously consistent with a history of severely reduced activity, but it provides no pathogenetic clues. The only other consistent observation was that, on the modified Gomori trichrome stain, the mitochondria appeared unusually prominent and distinct, although never amounting to the production of a "ragged-red" fiber. Histochemical stains were otherwise normal. We found no evidence of old or recent necrosis, no myophagocytosis, no inflammation, no focal mononuclear cell aggregates, and no interstitial fibrosis.

Ultrastructural Changes

Since the light microscopic examination of the biopsies had revealed no abnormalities, the ultrastructural findings were quite unexpected. Comparison with the surgical control group (Fig. 9-1) revealed mitochondrial changes in about 70% of the patients with CFS. In the subsarcolemmal region, the mitochondria were present in large aggregates of about two to three times the normal number and showed a range of sizes. Most were about twice normal size but some were considerably more, as much as 7 to 8 times normal. The majority retained the usual oval shape but a minority were pleomorphic. The most striking change was that from 50 to 100% of these organelles showed a very distinctive internal structure with an appearance of compartmentalization, apparently produced by branching and fusion of the cristae (Figs. 9-2, 9-3). At the sites of this branching and fusion, the cristae lost their usual parallel arrangement (Fig. 9-4). The picture was usually regular and uniform with compartments all approximately the same size. No zigzag or concentric cristae were seen. The intermyofibrillar mitochondria showed a similar increase in number with occasional sinuous or tortuous shapes present. Again, they were increased in size and showed proliferation of cristae to form compartments.

We then used the image analyzer to measure the total area of mitochondria in the subsarcolemmal and intermyofibrillar regions, and the perimeter of the compartments in the affected mitochondria, in the CFS patients and surgical controls. We found that compartmentalized mitochondria contained twice the area of normal mitochondria. Based on the presence of the compartments, therefore, the surface area of metabolically active membrane was increased by several times in the patients with CFS compared with controls.

The mitochondrial changes were most consistently seen in Type 1 fibers. Type 2 fibers showed recognizable atrophy with wrinkling of the sarcolemma and aggregates of organelles in the reduced sarcoplasm. Compartmentalization and pleomorphism were less apparent. Focal or total vacuolation of mitochondria was rare in either fiber type. A mild excess of lipid and glycogen was usually present. The lipid was in globules and was closely related to adjacent mitochondria. Similarly, occasional enlarged and compartmentalized mitochondria lay in lakes of glycogen granules. Finally, one or two patients showed focal myofibrillar

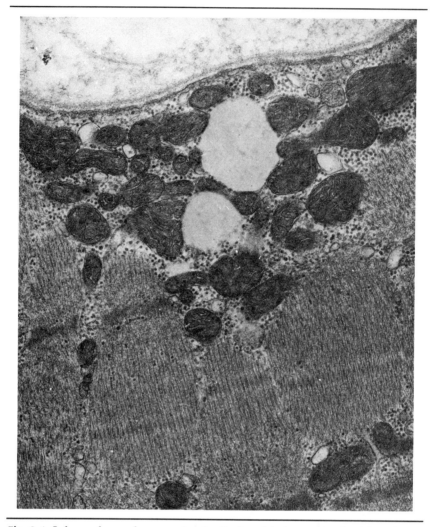

Fig. 9-1. Subsarcolemmal aggregate of mitochondria in a control subject shows cristae traversing the matrix. Two small lipid globules are present ($\times$ 30,000).

disruption associated with secondary lysosomes, but the rest revealed no evidence of muscle breakdown. Careful examination of the surgical control group revealed that occasional mitochondria showed compartmentalization, but they were not enlarged and their numbers did not exceed 5% of those present.

Medical Disease Controls

The group of patients with mixed connective tissue diseases showed, rarely, occasional fibers with severe mitochondrial abnormalities. These were grossly enlarged and sometimes demonstrated exactly the same striking compartmentalization as in the cases of CFS. These changes

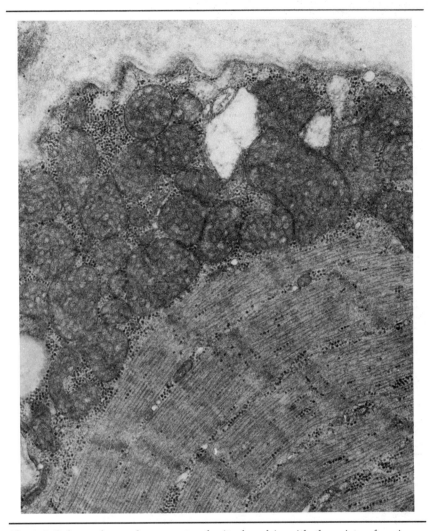

Fig. 9-2. Subsarcolemmal aggregate of mitochondria with the cristae forming compartments throughout the matrix in a patient with CFS ($\times$ 30,000).

were overshadowed, however, by evidence of fiber necrosis and regeneration, inflammation, and lysosomal debris. The patients with mitochondrial myopathies showed obvious abnormalities, as expected, with increase in number and size, pleomorphism, compartmentalization, and occasional zigzag cristae and crystalline inclusions.

IMPLICATIONS OF THE MUSCLE DEFECT IN CFS

The appearance of the compartmentalization in our CFS patients is similar to that described in the mitochondrial myopathies as "honeycomb-

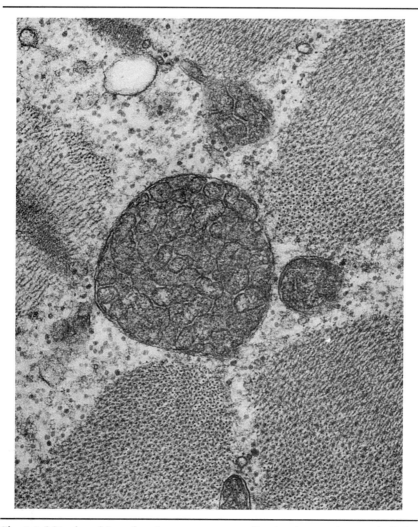

Fig. 9-3. Mitochondrion showing compartmentalization in a patient with CFS
(× 60,000).

ing" [13]. In the latter disorders, when structural abnormalities are
present, the mitochondria are more numerous, larger, and pleomorphic;
they develop abundant branched cristae, have an increased matrix, and
are surrounded by more and larger triglyceride droplets. Sometimes
crystalline or paracrystalline structures are seen [13]. In essence, all these
changes represent hyperplasia and can be interpreted as a compensatory
reactive process. They are not specific for any one enzyme defect but
are associated with dysfunction in oxidative phosphorylation and disorders of the respiratory chain [13]. The fact that similar, although less
severe features are present in CFS suggests that in this disorder also,

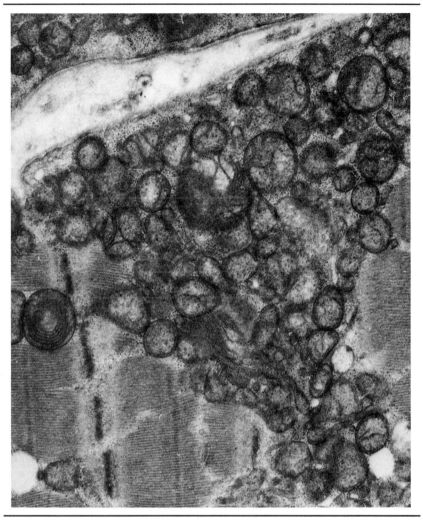

Fig. 9-4. Subsarcolemmal aggregate of mitochondria in a patient with mitochondrial myopathy, showing variation in size and number of cristae. Concentric cristae are present at one point ($\times$ 30,000).

there may be one or more functional defects with an attempt at compensation.

Fatigue, either induced or made worse by exertion, is the main characteristic of the mitochondrial myopathies, presumably because these mitochondria have an impaired capacity to generate high-energy phosphate bonds. Fatigue itself—the failure to sustain force or power output—may be central or peripheral in origin. Unlike the mitochondrial myopathies, in CFS there is undoubted evidence of central nervous system involvement so that a central component is likely [14], but the findings reported here suggest that there is also a peripheral lesion in the muscle.

Several studies have been carried out in CFS in an attempt to define the muscle lesions. Single-fiber electromyography has revealed myopathic features [7,15]. On the other hand, muscle performance, voluntary activation, twitch properties, and perceived effort were studied recently in 12 male patients with CFS compared to 13 healthy subjects [16]. No difference was found in motivation or perceived exertion between the two groups nor was there any difference in muscle activation, whether voluntary or electrically induced. The investigators concluded that neither poor motivation nor muscle contractile failure could account for the fatigue in these cases [16].

Magnetic resonance spectroscopy (MRS) has been used in the noninvasive investigation of metabolic muscle diseases. Most of the ATP required by muscle cells at rest is supplied by mitochondrial oxidative phosphorylation. During exercise, an increased demand for ATP is met mainly by an increase in this process. ^{31}P MRS can be used to monitor ATP, inorganic phosphate, phosphocreatine, and intracellular pH. In mitochondrial myopathies, the basic lesion appears to be impaired phosphorylation of adenosine diphosphate (ADP) to ATP. It is of great interest that a similar lesion has been reported in some cases of CFS [17].

Other biochemical studies have produced differing results: Depression of State 3 respiration rates with Site I and II substrates was found in two patients [18], but later studies revealed no evidence of mitochondrial or glycolytic abnormalities [19]. Other workers have recorded a reduced aerobic work capacity but considered this had a central cause [20].

Our finding of enteroviral genome in the muscle of 53% of patients with PFS has led us to postulate a chronic enteroviral infection [21]. Mitochondrial damage is associated with chronic Coxsackie infection in vitro [22]. Enteroviral genome has also been reported in another disease, polymyositis/dermatomyositis (PM/DM) [23]. It may be significant therefore that, apart from CFS, the other disease in which the mitochondria showed most compartments in our study was indeed PM/DM.

CONCLUSION

We have found structural mitochondrial changes in the muscle biopsies of 70% of a large group of patients with CFS. The abnormalities consisted of an increase in number and size, pleomorphism, and a characteristic appearance of compartmentalization due to branching and fusion of cristae. Using an image analyzer, we calculated that the total internal mitochondrial surface area was approximately twice that in the control groups. Together with the proliferation of mitochondrial membrane in the compartments, therefore, a greatly increased area of metabolically active membrane is present.

The work reported here suggests that there is muscle mitochondrial involvement in CFS, thus providing a possible explanation for the fatigue. We postulate that the lesions are associated with persistent enteroviral infection.

REFERENCES

1. Behan, P. O., Behan, W. M. H. Postviral fatigue syndrome. *CRC Crit. Rev. Neurobiol.* 4:157, 1988.
2. Ramsay, A. M. Epidemic neuromyasthenia 1955–1978. *Postgrad. Med. J.* 54:718, 1978.
3. Behan, P. O., Behan, W. M. H., Bell, E. J. The postviral fatigue syndrome: An analysis of the findings in 50 cases. *J. Infect.* 10:211, 1985.
4. Holmes, G. P., Kaplan, J. E., Gantz, N. M., et al. Chronic fatigue syndrome: A working case definition. *Ann. Intern. Med.* 108:387, 1988.
5. Sharpe, M. C., Archard, L. C., Banatvala, J. E., et al. A report—Chronic fatigue syndrome: Guidelines for research. *J. R. Soc. Med.* 84:118, 1991.
6. McEvedy, C. P., Beard, A. W. Royal Free Epidemic of 1955: A reconsideration. *Br. Med. J.* 1:7, 1970.
7. Jamal, G. A., Hansen, S. Postviral fatigue syndrome: Evidence for underlying organic disturbance in the muscle fibre. *Eur. Neurol.* 29:273, 1989.
8. Arnold, D. C., Radda, G. K., Bore, P. J., et al. Excessive intracellular acidosis of skeletal muscles on exercise in a patient with a postviral exhaustion/fatigue syndrome. *Lancet* 1:1367, 1984.
9. Arnold, D. C., Bore, P. J., Radda, G. K., et al. Enhanced neuromuscular acidosis during exercise by patients with the postviral exhaustion/fatigue syndrome. *Neurology* 35 (Suppl 1):165, 1985.
10. Behan, W. M. G., More, I. A. R., Behan, P. O. Mitochondrial abnormalities in the postviral fatigue syndrome. *Acta Neuropathol.* 83:61, 1991.
11. Dubowitz, V. The procedure of muscle biopsy and histological and histochemical stains and reactions. In *Muscle Biopsy* (2nd ed.). London: Bailliere Tindall, 1985. Pp. 3–40.
12. Cullen, M. J., Mastaglia, F. L. Pathological reactions of skeletal muscle. In F. L. Mastaglia and J. Walton (eds.). *Skeletal Muscle Pathology.* London: Churchill Livingstone, 1982. Pp. 88–139.
13. DiMauro, S., Bonilla, E., Zevioni, M., et al. Mitochondrial myopathies. *Ann. Neurol.* 17:521, 1985.
14. Behan, P. O., and Bakheit, A. M. O. Clinical spectrum of postviral fatigue syndrome. *Br. Med. Bull.* 47:795, 1991.
15. Jamal, G. A., and Hansen, S. Postviral fatigue syndrome: Evidence for underlying organic disturbance in the muscle fibre. *Eur. Neurol.* 29:273, 1989.
16. Lloyd, A. R., Gandevia, S. C., and Hales, J. P. Muscle performance, voluntary activation, twitch properties and perceived effort in normal subjects and patients with the chronic fatigue syndrome. *Brain* 114:85, 1991.
17. Wagenmakers, A. J. M., Kaur, N., Coukley, J. H., et al. Mitochondrial metabolism in myopathy and myalgia. *Adv. Myochem.* 1:219, 1987.
18. Byrne, E., Trounce, I., and Dennett, X. Chronic relapsing myalgia (postviral): Clinical, histological and biochemical studies. *Aust. N.Z. J. Med.* 15:305, 1985.
19. Byrne, E., and Trounce, I. Chronic fatigue and myalgia syndrome: Mito-

chondrial and glycolytic studies in skeletal muscle. *J. Neurol. Neurosurg. Psychiatry* 50:743, 1987.

20. Riley, M. S., O'Brien, C. J., McCluskey, D. R., et al. Aerobic work capacity in patients with chronic fatigue syndrome. *Br. Med. J.* 301:953, 1990.
21. Gow, J., Behan, W. M. H., Clements, G. B., et al. Enteroviral sequences detected by polymerase chain reaction in muscle biopsies of patients with postviral fatigue syndrome. *Br. Med. J.* 302:692, 1991.
22. Kandolf, B., Canu, A., Hofschneider, P. H. Coxsackie B3 virus can replicate in cultured human foetal heart cells and is inhibited by interferon. *J. Mol. Cell. Cardiol.* 17:167, 1985.
23. Bowles, N. E., Sewry, C. A., Dubowitz, V., et al. Dermatomyositis, polymyositis and Coxsackie B virus infection. *Lancet* 1:1004, 1987.

10

Harvey Moldofsky

Sleep and Chronic Fatigue Syndrome

Chronic debilitating fatigue, generalized musculoskeletal pain, cognitive complaints, depression, and sleep difficulties that follow a febrile illness have perplexed patients and their physicians for a long time. Over the past 100 years, various medical, neurologic, or psychiatric labels have been applied to this constellation of symptoms. In the absence of any specific incriminating etiologic agent, a working group of the Centers for Disease Control in the United States recently suggested the descriptive diagnostic term *chronic fatigue syndrome* (CFS) [1]. Similar symptoms are featured in fibromyalgia (fibrositis) syndrome [2]. The presumed link of the symptoms to an infectious agent has stimulated some investigators to search for a specific virus that causes the illness. Concurrently, others have chosen to assess patients for immunologic aberrations that are hypothesized to account for the continued ill health.

Although sleep difficulty has been documented to be a feature of the illness, generally speaking, little attention has been devoted to this symptom and to the contribution of the sleeping-waking brain to the fatigue, myalgia, and psychologic complaints in CFS. The purpose of this chapter is to review the evidence indicating that a dysfunction of the sleep-wake systems is associated with these complaints, expressed in both chronic fatigue and fibromyalgia syndromes. In particular, research has shown an intimate link of the circadian sleep-wake system to the immune system. The emergence of fatigue, myalgia, and psychologic distress occurs following disruption of slow wave non–rapid

141

eye movement (NREM) sleep, alteration in immune functions caused by infectious agents, or the administration of specific immunologically active peptides that affect sleep. These findings suggest that dysfunction of aspects of the sleep and immune systems is implicated in the symptoms.

DISORDERED SLEEP, FATIGUE, DIFFUSE MYALGIA, AND FEBRILE ILLNESS

The relationship of disordered sleep to acute febrile illness has been documented by physicians over the centuries. In his aphorisms, Hippocrates observed that "when sleep puts an end to delirium, it is a good sign" [3]. His observation implied that disordered sleep causes the delirium and that restoration of sleep cures the illness [4]. Contemporary sleep physiology research confirms this speculation. When Karacan et al. [5] artificially induced fever in human subjects with etiocholanolone and an endotoxin derivative of *Salmonella abortus equii,* the subjects complained of fitful and unrefreshing sleep, headache, and general malaise. Their sleep physiology studies showed frequent awakenings, even from slow-wave (stage 4) NREM sleep, and increased wake time during the fever. The appearance of stage 4 sleep was delayed. Overall, the sleep electroencephalogram (EEG) indicated an elevated arousal state with reduced stage 4, REM sleep, and dreaming. With recovery from the fever, normal sleep physiology recordings were accompanied by quiet and refreshing sleep.

The systemic effects of acute febrile illness include not only disturbed sleep but also malaise, fatigue, intellectual difficulties, diffuse myalgia, and headache. With some viral illnesses (e.g., influenza or infectious mononucleosis), these symptoms usually subside after the fever and acute effects of the disease resolve. Patients who complain of symptoms months or years after their acute febrile illness share many clinical and physiologic features with patients whose symptoms did not start with an infectious disease.

FATIGUE, DIFFUSE MYALGIA, AND UNREFRESHING SLEEP IN FIBROMYALGIA AND CFS

Theoretic Speculations

Chronic diffuse musculoskeletal pain, psychologic distress, and light, unrefreshing sleep in the absence of any evidence for a structural abnormality or known disease has been the source of considerable theoretic speculation over the past hundred years. Beard [6] attributed the poor sleep, fatigue, and myalgia to a functional disorder of the nervous system. Based on the assumption that the nervous system can be exhausted in a manner similar to the loss of electricity from a battery, he coined the term *neurasthenia*. Beard speculated that the industrial demands of Western civilization served to promote this common illness.

Patients who complained of the troublesome myalgia led some physicians to consider that an inflammatory rheumatologic disease could be the basis for the complaints. Gowers [7] speculated that "lumbago," "muscular rheumatism," or "brachial myalgia" was the result of inflammation of fibrous tissue. Initial pathologic reports proved promising [8], but the idea of specific inflammatory disease did not stand the test of subsequent investigations [9–11]. "Fibrositis" became a convenient label for the poorly understood complaints and was of little academic interest [12].

In the absence of a known physical cause, investigators focused on the likelihood that a specific psychologic disturbance—and not simply neurasthenia—was at the core of the fatigue, myalgia, and poor sleep. Various psychiatric diagnoses have been attributed to the disorder over the years, including "psychogenic rheumatism," "hysteria," "masked depression," and currently "somatoform pain disorder." Now somatoform pain disorder is being questioned [13]: The judgment of what constitutes excessive pain may be impossible; the underlying medical condition may not be detected; and even though the pain may be consistent with the medical condition, it may respond to psychotropic drugs or psychologic techniques. Equally, the same arguments can be made for the chronic fatigue and the poor sleep.

Physicians who noted these "flulike" symptoms to persist following a febrile illness provided a host of labels. Some names referred to a region or hospital where large groups of people were afflicted; others were based on presumed involvement of the nervous and muscular systems (postinfectious neuromyasthenia, myalgic encephalomyelitis). Recently, etiologic labels (e.g., chronic mononucleosis, Epstein-Barr virus disorder) have been displaced in favor of the descriptive label *chronic fatigue syndrome* [1]. Likewise, "fibrositis" has been replaced with the descriptive term *fibromyalgia* [14]. In both populations, the research shows that a syndrome characterized by persistent unrefreshing sleep, chronic fatigue, diffuse myalgia, and psychologic distress is influenced by a disturbance in the sleeping-waking brain.

Common Clinical Features

As shown in Table 10-1, Goldenberg [2] reported that fibromyalgia and CFS share many similar clinical features. A majority of the patients are women approximately 40 years old. Eighty percent or more of patients in both diagnostic groups describe fatigue, myalgias and arthralgias, recurrent headache, and sleep disturbances. Similarly, in their review of fibromyalgia patients who shared the same diagnostic criteria as pa-

Table 10-1. Demographic and clinical features (%) of fibromyalgia and CFS[a]

	Fibromyalgia (N = 350)	CFS (N = 200)
Female (%)	87	79
Mean age (yr)	43	38
Fatigue	90	97
Myalgias, arthralgias	100	85
Recurrent headache	90	83
Sleep disturbances	95	93
Morning stiffness	95	63
Irritable bowel syndrome	80	63
Numbness, tingling	85	70
Raynaud's phenomenon	10	41
Depression, mood changes	72	78

[a]Fibromyalgia patients of Goldenberg and CFS patients of Komaroff (from Goldenberg [2]).

tients with CFS, Yunus and co-workers [14] and Wallace et al. [15] showed a predominance of fatigue, myalgias, arthralgias, and poor sleep. These symptoms paralleled clinical data obtained from their review of the scientific literature on patients diagnosed with CFS or myalgic encephalomyelitis. On the other hand, Wysenbeek et al. [16] showed that while there were similarities in symptoms, only seven of their 33 patients with fibromyalgia fulfilled the Holmes et al. [1] criteria for CFS. The poor sleep, fatigue, number of painful sites, and tender points in specific anatomic regions were found not to be related to personality disturbances in fibromyalgia patients [14].

SLEEP PHYSIOLOGY AND THE NONRESTORATIVE SLEEP SYNDROME

Sleep physiology studies of patients with fibromyalgia showed an alpha (7.5–11.0 Hz) EEG anomaly during NREM sleep that was related to patients' unrefreshing sleep and overnight increase in muscle tenderness [17]. This sleep anomaly was interpreted as an indicator of an arousal disorder within sleep and the subjective experience of nonrestorative sleep. Consistent with this notion, Anch et al. [18] showed that fibromyalgia patients had more alpha EEG sleep, were more vigilant during sleep, and had more fatigue, sleepiness, and pain than normal healthy controls.

Such a constellation of altered sleep physiology and symptoms comprises a nonrestorative sleep syndrome. A series of research studies have shown that factors that disturb sleep physiology—such as psychologic distress, noxious environmental disturbance, primary sleep disorders, or inflammatory joint disease—contribute to this syndrome: The alpha EEG sleep anomaly, diffuse myalgia, fatigue, and emotional distress were found in patients following an emotionally distressing but not physically injurious industrial or automobile accident [19]. The sleep anomaly and symptoms were experimentally produced by noise disruption of stage 4 NREM sleep in normal sedentary people, but not in a small group of physically fit runners [20]. Fragmented sleep with periodic limb movements [21,22] or sleep apnea [23] has been found in patients with fibromyalgia symptoms. Based on the presumption that painful inflamed points in patients with rheumatoid arthritis would disturb sleep, abnormal sleep physiology findings would be related to the joint and muscle complaints and exhaustion that characterize the morning symptoms. Indeed, such patients showed the alpha EEG sleep anomaly, increased weakness, articular and nonarticular tenderness, and an overnight reduction in energy [24]. In addition to the alpha EEG sleep anomaly, both Mahowald and colleagues [25] and Lavie et al. [26] reported that some rheumatoid patients had sleep-related periodic limb movements and apneas.

The similarity of sleep physiology patterns and symptoms in patients with fibromyalgia and CFS has been shown in two studies. In the first, sleep physiology and symptoms were compared in patients with fibromyalgia that followed upon a severe febrile illness, patients who did not attribute their symptoms to any infectious illness, and normal control subjects. Both the postfebrile and nonfebrile groups showed similar increased alpha EEG ratings during their sleep in comparison to the normal controls. Likewise, the patient groups reported more musculoskeletal pain before and after sleep [27]. Recently, in a study that compared CFS patients with normal subjects, Whelton, Salit, and Moldofsky [28] showed that the patients had more difficulty falling asleep, spent less time asleep, had reduced REM sleep, and demonstrated greater alpha EEG activity during NREM sleep. Three of our 14 patients also had other specific sleep abnormalities: two had sleep apnea and the third experienced periodic limb movements during sleep. Such primary sleep disorders were also reported by Krupp and Mendelson [29].

Like fibromyalgia patients, our chronic fatigue patients complained of diffuse myalgia and had more tender points than normal controls [28]. Despite the fact that most patients expressed an increased need for sleep, they were not shown to be physiologically hypersomnolent during the course of the day. The lack of excessive daytime sleepiness in these patients sharply contrasts with the EEG demonstration of sleepiness in 10 patients following infectious mononucleosis and two following Guillain-Barré syndrome [30].

RELATIONSHIP OF THE IMMUNE SYSTEM TO SLEEP AND SYMPTOMS

Research studies demonstrate that aspects of cytokines and cellular immune functions are linked to sleep-wake physiology. Certain cytokines and products of infectious agents have sleep-promoting effects in animals. These experiments and the clinical observation that disordered sleep, chronic fatigue, and diffuse myalgia are induced by administration of some of these cytokines suggest that a disturbance in sleep-wake immune functions may provide a pathophysiologic link to the symptoms of chronic fatigue and fibromyalgia syndromes.

The Immune System and Sleep-Wake Physiology

The immune system is fundamentally involved in guarding against disease but is also important in bodily regulatory functions. Of special interest is interleukin-1 (IL-1), a polypeptide cytokine classified into IL-1α and IL-1β subtypes. It is synthesized by a variety of activated cells, including astroglial cells of the brain, and is considered to be a key factor in homeostatic mechanisms. IL-1 acts via the central nervous system to induce fever and the acute phase inflammatory response. This peptide induces the release of several hypothalamic and pituitary hormones including endorphins, corticotropin-releasing factor, adrenocorticotropic hormone, and somatostatin [31]. IL-1 is involved in numerous central and peripheral biologic activities that involve various cellular and humoral aspects of the immune system. It has been studied in a variety of inflammatory and malignant diseases [32].

Because of the central importance of IL-1 to the immune system and the observation that it promotes slow wave sleep in animals [33], we studied changes in IL-1 activity and related immune and endocrine functions over the sleep-wake cycle. We showed that maximum plasma IL-1- and IL-2-like activities occurred during nocturnal sleep in humans [27]; similarly, IL-1 activity in the cerebrospinal fluid was increased during sleep versus wakefulness in cats [34]. These data are consistent with the observation that IL-1 is not only related to slow wave sleep in animals, but may—along with other peptides (e.g., factor S, muramyl dipeptide, vasoactive intestinal peptide, prostaglandin D_2, interferon-α_2, tumor necrosis factor [33], and Il-2 [35]—be one of the key mediating agents involved in promoting sleep. While microinjections of IL-1 into various basal forebrain regions indicated separate sites for sleep and fever, the somnogenic sites of action for IL-1 and muramyl peptides are unknown [36]. Kreuger and Johannsen [33] have suggested that the various immunologically active peptides interact in a complex fashion with different hypothalamic-pituitary hormones in regulating the delicate balance of sleep-wake functions.

In fact, cellular immune functions appear to be associated with the sleep-wake cycle. B cell lymphocyte responsiveness assessed with the in vitro pokeweed mitogen (PWM) test showed greater activity during nocturnal sleep, while plasma cortisol declined. Natural killer (NK) cell activity precipitously declined following sleep onset. The reason for this diminished activity is unknown, but may relate to either reduced function of NK cells or their disappearance from the circulation with distribution in the tissues to perform immune surveillance and lysis of pathogenic cells. Similar functional changes have been observed in women during the low-progesterone phase of the menstrual cycle. However, during the high-progesterone phase, stage 4 sleep was delayed and reduced, as were NK cell activities [37].

These observations from human and animal studies are consistent with the hypothesis that sleep-related immune functions are involved in the physiologic restorative function of sleep. Therefore, disruption of normal overnight sleep physiology would be expected to cause alteration in immune functions and give rise to nonrestorative sleep symptoms. Alternatively, alteration in the immune functions would be associated with disturbances in sleep physiology and nonrestorative sleep symptoms.

The Effects of Sleep Disruption on Immune Functions and Behavior

Sleep deprivation has been used to determine the effects of altered sleep physiology on psychologic and physiologic functions. Sleep deprivation is well known to cause sleepiness, fatigue, negative mood, and impairment in a variety of intellectual functions. Prolonged wakefulness has also been shown to affect the immune system.

The disturbances in psychologic function as the result of sleep deprivation are reminiscent of the psychologic difficulties reported by patients with CFS. That is, with prolonged wakefulness not only is there sleepiness, fatigue, and emotional distress, but also progressive cognitive and temporal disorganization with impaired performance on vigilance and memory tasks. Initially, subjects experience difficulty thinking of words. They may make mistakes about time. Often they have problems maintaining concentration, especially with tedious, repetitive tasks. They become forgetful. Horne [38] in his analysis of the function of sleep argues that the impairments are reversible with normal sleep. He claims slow-wave sleep is obligatory to the restitution of intellectual impairment that results from sleep deprivation [38].

Several studies have shown alterations in immune functions following sleep deprivation. A study of normal subjects following 72 hours of sleep deprivation showed reduced phagocytosis by polymorphonuclear granulocytes, increased interferon production by lymphocytes, and increased plasma cortisol [39]. A study of the effects of 48 hours of wakefulness showed a reduced phytohemagglutinin (PHA) mitogen response [40]. These studies were flawed by their reliance on a single morning blood sample and the emotional stress of the experimental procedure [38].

Assessments of serial blood samples in a study of the effects of 40 hours of wakefulness showed dramatic changes in plasma IL-1 and IL-2 activities and aspects of cellular immune functions. The rise of nocturnal PWM response that occurs during the normal baseline 24-hour wake-sleep cycle was delayed by sleep deprivation. PHA mitogen response showed no change with the sleep deprivation. The activity of NK cells did not decline during nocturnal sustained wakefulness, as it had during baseline sleep, but NK activity was continually reduced throughout the period of resumed nocturnal sleep. Night-time plasma IL-1 and IL-2 activities were higher during the early hours of the night of sleep deprivation compared to baseline and resumed sleep. The changes observed in these immune functions during sleep deprivation were unrelated to changes in diurnal cortisol, indicating that they were not caused by any physiologic stress inherent in the procedures. Repeated behavioral and performance assessments showed that negative mood, sleepiness, and fatigue correlated with PWM responses. Reaction time and logical reasoning were directly related to PHA response and to plasma IL-1 activity.

A subsequent study of the effect of 64 hours of wakefulness in five subjects showed greater disorder in 24-hour patterns of mitogen functional assays and NK cell activity. Even with a single night of sleep, patients failed to return to their normal baseline patterns. Furthermore, two subjects developed upper respiratory infections within the week after the study. One of them experienced asthmatic symptoms for the first time. Such anecdotal observations do not prove that respiratory symptoms result from vulnerability to disease caused by disruption in integrated sleep-related functions involving the immune system. However, this idea is supported by experimental studies showing that sleep-deprived mice previously immunized against influenza virus did not clear the virus from their lungs when challenged with the infectious agent. In contrast, immunized and challenged mice that slept normally showed no evidence of virus in their lungs [41].

Effects of Altered Immune Functions on Sleep and Behavior

Commonly, alterations in immune functions occur as the result of bacterial or viral agents. Sleepiness, fatigue, negative mood, and intellectual difficulties are topical features of a febrile illness. Recently, Krueger and colleagues [42] showed an intimate link between infectious agents and the sleeping brain. Inoculation of viable or heat-killed *Staphylococcus aureus* and *Escherichia coli* enhanced slow-wave sleep and increased body temperature in rabbits. The digested bacterial product of macrophages had a similar effect, as did lipid A and specific muramyl peptides that are products of bacterial cell walls. Similarly, polyriboinosinic : polyribocytidylic acid (Poly I : C), a synthetic double-stranded RNA that provokes the fever and systemic symptoms of a viral illness, has somnogenic effects if administered intravenously or into the cerebral ventricles of rabbits. These infectious agents appear to have the capacity to alter sleep via IL-1, several other immunologically active peptides, and neuroendocrine hormonal mechanisms [42].

In human immunodeficiency virus (HIV) infection, 29% of patients showed fibromyalgia symptoms [43]. Patients who have been exposed to HIV infection but do not exhibit symptoms also have altered sleep physiology. They show a delay in sleep onset, the alpha EEG sleep anomaly, and increases in slow-wave sleep, total NREM periods, and awakenings during sleep [44]. In addition to HIV, fibromyalgia has been associated with other viral infections including Coxsackie B [45] and parvovirus; the latter has been accompanied by the alpha EEG sleep anomaly [46].

Not only are these various viral agents associated with symptoms of fibromyalgia or CFS, but the symptoms have been induced with immunologic peptides that influence sleep. Interferon-α given to hepatitis carriers caused fatigue, cognitive dysfunction [47], and diffuse myalgia and malaise. IL-2 employed in the treatment of cancer has been shown to produce severe cognitive impairment and an influenza-like syndrome. Patients complain of decreased energy, fatigue, anorexia, malaise, reduced interest, sleep disturbances [48], and diffuse musculoskeletal symptoms similar to those of fibromyalgia [15]. Although changes in interferon-γ production by peripheral mononuclear cells have not been demonstrated in patients with CFS [49], production of interferon-α was found to be excessive [50]. Moreover, serum IL-2 was elevated in patients with chronic fatigue disorder [51]. The exacerbation of fatigue, myalgia, and sleep symptoms provoked by physical exercise may be partly the result of increased IL-1 and interferon activity with acute phase response that produces skeletal muscle proteolysis [52]. Therefore, disordered regulation of the cytokines interferon-α, IL-1, and IL-2 likely provokes alterations in immune and sleep-wake systems that accompany many of the symptoms attributed to chronic fatigue or fibromyalgia disorders.

CONCLUSION

Various research studies show that the amalgam of disordered sleep physiology, chronic fatigue, diffuse myalgia, and cognitive and behavioral symptoms comprises a nonrestorative sleep syndrome that may follow a febrile illness, as in the chronic fatigue disorder. Where rheumatic complaints are prominent, such a constellation of disturbed sleep physiology and symptoms also characterizes the fibromyalgia disorder. In contrast to CFS, fibromyalgia has been shown to be associated with a variety of initiating or perpetuating factors such as psychologically distressing events, primary sleep disorders (e.g., sleep apnea, periodic limb movement disorder), inflammatory rheumatic disease, as well as an acute febrile illness. The chronic fatigue and fibromyalgia syndromes have similar disordered sleep physiology, which shows features of an arousal disturbance within NREM sleep with increased nocturnal vigilance that accompanies the usually light and unrefreshing sleep experience.

Aspects of cytokine and cellular immune functions are shown to be related to the sleep-wake system. The research suggests a reciprocal relationship of the immune and sleep-wake systems. Interference with either the immune system (e.g., by a viral agent, cytokines such as interferon-α or IL-2) or the sleeping-waking brain system (e.g., sleep deprivation) will affect the other with accompanying sleep abnormalities, fatigue, diffuse myalgia, and behavioral symptoms that are features in CFS.

REFERENCES

1. Holmes, G. P., Kaplan, J. E., Grantz, N. M., et al. Chronic fatigue syndrome: A working case definition. *Ann. Intern. Med.* 108:387, 1988.
2. Goldenberg, D. L. Fibromyalgia and its relation to chronic fatigue syndrome, viral illness and immune abnormalities. *J. Rheumatol.* 16 (Suppl. 19):91, 1989.
3. Hippocrates. Translated by F. Adams. Chicago: *Encyclopaedia Britannica*, 1952.
4. Lipowski, Z. J. Delirium, acute brain failure in man. Springfield, Ill.: Charles C. Thomas, 1980. P. 8.
5. Karacan, I., Wolff, S. M., Williams, R. L., et al. The effects of fever on sleep and dream patterns. *Psychosomatics* 9:331, 1968.
6. Beard, G. M. *American Nervousness: Its Causes and Consequences*. New York: G. P. Putnam, 1881.
7. Gowers, W. R. Lumbago and its analogues. *Br. Med. J.* 1:117, 1904.
8. Stockman, R. The causes, pathology and treatment of chronic rheumatism. *Edinb. Med. J.* 15:107, 1904.
9. Abel, O., Seibert, A. J., and Earp, R. Fibrositis. *J. Missouri Med. Assoc.* 36:435, 1939.
10. Collins, D. H. Fibrositis and infection. *Ann. Rheum. Dis.* 2:114, 1940.
11. Slocumb, C. G. Fibrositis. *Clinics* 2:169, 1943.
12. Bennett, R. M. Fibrositis: Evolution of an enigma. *J. Rheumatol.* 13:676, 1986.
13. Frances, A., First, M. B., Pincuslt, A., and Widiger, T. A. DSM IV Option Book: Work in Progress (7/1/91). Task Force on DSM IV. Washington, D.C.: American Psychiatric Association, 1991. P. I 9.
14. Yunus, M., Masi, A. T., Calabro, J. J., et al. Primary fibromyalgia (fibrositis): Clinical study of 50 patients and matched controls. *Arthritis Rheum.* 11:151, 1981.
15. Wallace, D. J., Peter, J. B., Bowman, R. L., et al. Fibromyalgia, cytokines, fatigue syndromes and immune regulation. In J. R. Fricton and E. Awad (eds.). *Advances in Pain Research and Therapy* (Vol. 17, Chap. 18). New York: Raven, 1990. Pp. 277–287.
16. Wysenbeek, A. J., Shapira, Y., and Leibovici, L. Primary fibromyalgia and the chronic fatigue syndrome. *Rheumatol. Int.* 10:227, 1991.
17. Moldofsky, H., Scarisbrick, P., England, R., and Smythe, H. Musculoskeletal symptoms and non-REM sleep disturbance in patients with "fibrositis syndrome" and healthy subjects. *Psychosom. Med.* 34:341, 1975.
18. Anch, A. M., Lue, F. A., MacLean, A. W., and Moldofsky, H. Sleep phys-

iology and psychological aspects of fibrositis (fibromyalgia syndrome). *Can. J. Psychol.* 45:179, 1991.
19. Saskin, P., Moldofsky, H., and Lue, F. A. Sleep and posttraumatic rheumatic pain modulation disorder (fibrositis syndrome). *Psychosom. Med.* 48:319, 1986.
20. Moldofsky, H., and Scarisbrick, P. Induction of neurasthenic musculoskeletal pain syndrome by selective sleep stage deprivation. *Psychosom. Med.* 38:35, 1976.
21. Moldofsky, H., Tullis, C., Lue, F. A., et al. Sleep-related myoclonus in rheumatic pain modulation disorder (fibrositis syndrome) and in excessive daytime somnolence. *Psychosom. Med.* 46:145, 1984.
22. Hamm, C., Derman, S., et al. Sleep parameters in fibrositis/fibromyalgia syndrome. *Arthritis Rheum.* 32(4):S70, 1989.
23. Molony, R. R., MacPeck, D. M., Schiffman, P. L., et al. Sleep, sleep apnea and the fibromyalgia syndrome. *J. Rheumatol.* 13:797, 1986.
24. Moldofsky, H., Lue, F. A., and Smythe, H. A. Alpha EEG sleep and morning symptoms in rheumatoid arthritis. *J. Rheumatol.* 10:373, 1983.
25. Mahowald, M. W., Mahowald, M. L., Bundlie, S. R., and Ytterberg, S. R. Sleep fragmentation in rheumatoid arthritis. *Arthritis Rheum.* 32:974, 1989.
26. Lavie, P., Nahir, M., Lorber, M., and Scharf, Y. Nonsteroidal antiinflammatory drug therapy in rheumatoid arthritis. *Arthritis Rheum.* 34:655, 1991.
27. Moldofsky, H., Saskin, P., and Lue, F. A. Sleep and symptoms in fibrositis syndrome after a febrile illness. *J. Rheumatol.* 15:1701, 1988.
28. Whelton, D. L., Salit, I., and Moldofsky, H. Sleep, Epstein-Barr virus infection, musculoskeletal pain, and depressive symptoms in chronic fatigue syndrome. *J. Rheumatol.* (In press.)
29. Krupp, L. B., and Mendelson, W. B. Sleep characteristics in chronic fatigue syndrome. *Sleep Res.* 19:333, 1990.
30. Guilleminault, C., and Mondini, S. Mononucleosis and chronic daytime sleepiness: A long term follow-up study. *Arch. Intern. Med.* 146:1333, 1986.
31. Dinarello, C. A. Biology of interleukin-1. *FASEB J.* 2:108, 1988.
32. Platonias, L. C., and Vogelzang, N. J. Interleukin-1: Biology, pathophysiology and clinical prospects. *Am. J. Med.* 89:621, 1990.
33. Krueger, J. M., and Johannsen, L. Bacterial products, cytokines and sleep. In A. Lenmark, T. Dyrberg, L. Terenius, and B. Hokfelt (eds.) *Molecular Mimicry in Health and Disease.* New York: Elsevier, 1988. Pp. 35–46.
34. Lue, F. A., Bail, M., Jephthah-Ochola, J., et al. Sleep and cerebrospinal fluid interleukin-1-like activity in the cat. *Int. J. Neurosci.* 42:179, 1988.
35. Nistico, G., and De Sarro, G. Is interleukin 2 a neuromodulator in the brain. *Trends Neurosci.* 14:146, 1991.
36. Walter, J. S., Meyers, P., and Krueger, J. M. Microinjections of interleukin-1 into brain: Separation of sleep and fever responses. *Physiol. Behavior* 45:169, 1989.
37. Moldofsky, H., Lue, F., Shahal, B., et al. Circadian immune functions & the menstrual cycle in healthy women. *Sleep Res.* 20A:552, 1991.
38. Horne, J. *The Functions of Sleep in Humans and Other Mammals.* Oxford, England: Oxford University Press, 1988.
39. Palmblad, J., Cantell, K., Strander, H., et al. Stressor exposure and immunological response in man: Interferon producing capacity and phagocytosis. *J. Psychosom. Res.* 20:193, 1976.
40. Palmblad, J., Petrini, B., Wasserman, J., and Akerstedt, T. Lymphocyte and granulocyte reactions during sleep deprivation. *Psychosom. Med.* 41:273, 1977.
41. Brown, R., Price, R. J., King, M. G., and Husband, A. J. Interleukin-1 beta and muramyl dipeptide can prevent decreased antibody response associated with sleep deprivation. *Brain Behav. Immun.* 3(4):320, 1989.

42. Krueger, J. M., Obal, F., Opp, M., et al. Putative sleep neuromodulators. In J. Montplaisir and R. Godbout (eds.). *Sleep and Biological Rhythms: Basic Mechanisms and Applications to Psychiatry* (Chap. 10). New York: Oxford University Press, 1990.
43. Buskila, D., Gladman, D. D., Langevitz, P., et al. Fibromyalgia in human immunodeficiency virus infection. *J. Rheumatol.* 17:1202, 1990.
44. Norman, S. E., Chediak, A., Kiel, M., et al. HIV infection and sleep: Follow up studies. *Sleep Res.* 19:339, 1990.
45. Nash, P., Chard, M., and Hazleman, B. Chronic Coxsackie B infection mimicking primary fibromyalgia. *J. Rheumatol.* 16:1506, 1989.
46. Leventhal, L. J., Naides, S. J., and Freundlich, B. Fibromyalgia and parvovirus infection. *Arthritis Rheum.* 34:1319, 1991.
47. McDonald, E. M., Mann, A. H., and Thomas, H. C. Interferons as mediators of psychiatric morbidity: An investigation in a trial of recombinant alpha interferon in hepatitis-B carriers. *Lancet* 2:1175, 1987.
48. Denicoff, K. D., Rubinow, D. R., Papa, M. Z., et al. The neuropsychiatric effects of treatment with interleukin-2 and lymphokine activated killer cells. *Ann. Intern. Med.* 107:293, 1987.
49. Morte, S., Castilla, A., Civeira, M. P., et al. Gamma-interferon and chronic fatigue syndrome. *Lancet* 2:623, 1988.
50. Lever, A. M. C., Lewis, D. M., Bannister, B. A., et al. Interferon production in post viral fatigue syndrome (letter). *Lancet* 2:101, 1988.
51. Cheney, P. R., Dorman, S. E., and Bell, D. S. Interleukin-2 and the chronic fatigue syndrome. *Ann. Intern. Med.* 110:321, 1989.
52. Cannon, J. B., Fielding, R. A., Fiatarone, M. A., et al. Increased interleukin 1β in human skeletal muscle after exercise. *Am. J. Physiol.* 257:R451, 1989.

11

Loren A. Rolak

Fatigue and Multiple Sclerosis

Multiple sclerosis (MS) causes exacerbating and remitting episodes of demyelination in the brain and spinal cord. It injures the myelin sheath, the modified membrane that insulates neurons and enhances their capacity for electrical conduction. Attacks on the myelin—inflammatory episodes that presumably have an autoimmune basis—often produce damage sufficient to destroy nerve conduction, resulting in paralysis, blindness, or other focal neurologic deficits. Striking primarily young adults, MS is the most common disabling neurologic disease between the ages of 20 and 40, affecting nearly 250,000 Americans [1].

Fatigue is a frequent and serious symptoms of MS. In a recent study of 656 MS patients, 78% complained of fatigue, 69% experienced it every day, and 22% suffered disruption of their daily activities [2]. Similar results came from a carefully controlled survey showing that 88% of MS patients felt fatigue and in 28% it was their most severe symptom [3]. In another survey, of 100 British MS patients, 47% reported significant fatigue within the past month [4]. In the United States, the National Multiple Sclerosis Society recently evaluated 839 patients who had had MS for longer than 10 years but suffered only minimal impairments. In this group of mildly affected patients, fatigue was the most frequently reported current symptom [5].

Fatigue in MS is not only common, but also severe. Forty percent of MS patients list it as the most serious symptom of their disease [6], and it causes at least temporary disability in up to 75% of patients [1]. Fatigue forces substantial adaptations in the working environment, and the British MS Society found it to be the most important symptom leading to unemployment among victims of the disease [1].

Physicians and laymen alike are usually surprised that fatigue causes so much disability in a disease more commonly associated with such devastating symptoms as blindness, paralysis, and ataxia. Many doctors do not accept fatigue as a legitimate symptom. This occurs, in part, because fatigue can be normal (like insomnia) and because it cannot be measured well by tangible parameters (such as test scores) [4]. Also, there are no generally accepted criteria for defining fatigue or differentiating it from depression, weakness, and other accompaniments of MS. The experience of fatigue is difficult to communicate to others and is thus often attributed to neurosis [7]. It is one of the least understood symptoms in MS.

DEFINITION

Various studies have described MS fatigue in different terms. Researchers as well as patients themselves disagree about precisely what constitutes MS fatigue. Seventy-six percent of patients in one survey felt their fatigue was different from anything they had ever experienced prior to MS, and was not related to normal sensations of tiredness or lack of energy [6]. Another study agreed that the sensation of extreme tiredness in MS has a quality all its own, but found that it resembles the fatigue that occurs in influenza [7]. Some patients conceptualize a fixed quantity of energy that runs out over a period of time (suggesting that pacing one's activities will decrease fatigue) [4]. The fatigue of MS is often described as a sense of lassitude and lack of the physical energy necessary to perform tasks—not as a sleepiness, boredom, or depression [3].

A study specifically designed to characterize the fatigue of MS found that the most useful way of differentiating it from the normal fatigue occasionally experienced by everyone is by its effect on activities of daily living [3]. The fatigue of MS actually prevents physical functioning in 87% of patients, whereas none of the normal controls reported that fatigue could physically prevent them from performing tasks. Walking and standing are the activities most affected by fatigue in MS [8]. The fatigue primarily interferes with physical rather than mental activity [8]. Another useful distinguishing feature is that the fatigue of MS is usually worsened by heat, and is very sensitive to increases in temperature [3] (Table 11-1).

The two most important conditions mimicking fatigue in MS are sedation from drugs and depression [1]. Many of the drugs frequently given to patients with MS can cause sedation, which may be confused with fatigue. These include antispastic agents such as baclofen and diazepam,

Table 11-1. Differences between the fatigue
of multiple sclerosis and normal fatigue

The fatigue of MS resembles normal fatigue in that it is:
1. Often characterized as a need to rest
2. Accompanied by decreased motivation and patience
3. Worse at the end of the day
4. Aggravated by exercise and depression
5. Improved by rest and positive experiences

The fatigue of MS differs from normal fatigue in that it:
1. Interferes with physical functioning and activities of daily living
2. Is worsened by heat
3. Comes on easily

Source: Adapted from Krupp et al. [3].

tricyclic medications, anticonvulsants, and treatments for tremor. Depression, a common accompaniment of MS, can produce apathy and a sense of fatigue that resembles the true fatigue of MS.

MS fatigue occurs daily, either continuously or intermittently. For some patients, unremitting fatigue lingers as a constant, chronic presence; but most patients describe it as more episodic, generally peaking in the late afternoon and lasting a few hours [4,9]. Such patients often think of episodes of fatigue as resembling short exacerbations of their MS [2,6]. Certainly, fatigue can come and go, like any MS symptom.

Fatigue correlates poorly with any other physical or emotional aspect of MS [1]. It afflicts some patients who suffer little other neurologic disability, while in others it worsens just before and during a relapse [10]. It can appear as a prodrome to an exacerbation [2]. Indeed, fatigue can be the first symptom of MS: One study found it predated all other symptoms in 31% of patients [3]. Although depression occurs more commonly among MS patients than controls, there is no strong relationship between depression and fatigue in MS [3].

Fatigue can worsen from mental as well as physical activity, but the problem of objectively measuring fatigue makes it difficult to analyze this effect. One study measured simple reaction times in MS patients, then gave them an exhausting 4-hour neuropsychologic evaluation and retested them. There was no deterioration in their reaction time after this mental effort, even among patients who complained of fatigue [11].

MECHANISM OF FATIGUE

A number of different mechanisms have been postulated to explain the excessive fatigue found among MS patients, but none have been universally endorsed. A widely accepted theory accounts for fatigue as a simple increase in energy demands caused by neurologic disability. The metabolic "cost of walking," as measured by oxygen consumption, is 3 or 4 times greater in MS patients than controls, an increased requirement that poses an extra burden on the cardiorespiratory system [12]. When MS patients exercise on a treadmill, the most frequent reason for halting is a sense of generalized fatigue. The increased cardiorespiratory and metabolic demands could at least partly account for the symptom of fatigue in MS. This increased cost of exercise also occurs after a spinal cord injury or hemiparetic stroke, and accompanies lower extremity difficulties. But leg spasticity, rather than weakness, correlates best with fatigue. For example, patients with myopathies can have considerable weakness, but because they do not have spasticity, their metabolic demands are not increased and so they do not experience much fatigue. This theory predicts that physical therapy and antispastic agents should help reduce metabolic demands, and hence minimize fatigue in MS. Some authorities discount this explanation, however, because many MS patients with fatigue have no lower extremity spasticity (or weakness). Also, some diseases, such as the postpolio syndrome, characteristically cause considerable fatigue but no spasticity.

A similar study analyzed lower extremity function and fatigue in patients with spastic paraparesis, most of whom had MS [13]. Tetanic electrical stimulation of nerves produced muscle contraction that was weak and that fatigued quickly with repetitive stimulation. Repeated muscle contraction also produced lower phosphocreatine and pH levels in patients than in controls. The authors suggested that impaired function of the muscles of patients with upper motor neuron lesions may contribute to their feelings of excessive fatigue.

In addition to muscle problems, some patients with MS have defects in neuromuscular transmission and respond physiologically in a fashion similar to that seen in myasthenia gravis. This could explain at least some of their symptoms of fatigability [14].

Nerve conduction abnormalities within the central nervous system could account for fatigue as well. Demyelinated nerves do not transmit action potentials efficiently, largely because of altered ionic flow across sodium and potassium channels. Some authors speculate that these weakened action potentials could translate into a clinical symptom of fatigue [1].

Fatigue may also result from poor physical fitness and deconditioning in MS patients, as it does in some patients with traumatic spinal cord injury. A recent study showed respiratory muscle weakness and increased resting heart rates in MS patients, and concluded that fatigue was due to the high energy cost of physical activity such as walking, combined with poor conditioning and altered cardiovascular control. Theoretically, then, fatigue could be lessened by physical training [15].

Autonomic dysfunction may contribute to fatigue [16]. Sympathetic activity is impaired in many MS patients, which correlates with a feeling of fatigue. Whether the relative excess of parasympathetic tone directly accounts for the fatigue, or whether some other mechanism operates to produce it, is not yet clear.

Other studies have examined an autoimmune basis for fatigue. Experiments with interleukin-2 revealed that one of its primary side effects is fatigue and loss of energy. Elevated interleukin-2 levels, a common finding in many MS patients, have been blamed for producing fatigue [17]. However, in a study of eight patients with MS who complained of severe fatigue, interleukin-2 serum levels were identical to those in normal controls, casting doubt on any correlation between interleukin-2 and fatigue [18].

THERAPY

Amantadine

Because the mechanism of fatigue is not clear, its treatment, too, is uncertain. Amantadine was the first drug, and is still one of the few, proved effective for treating the fatigue of MS. This benefit was discovered serendipitously when patients placed on amantadine as prophylaxis against influenza spontaneously reported a diminution in their fatigue. This clinical observation was tested in prospective controlled trials that verified its validity. A preliminary double-blind controlled trial of amantadine in 32 patients found 62% of them better compared with 22% in the placebo group [6]. A follow-up multicenter prospective randomized double-blind trial in 115 patients, using a visual analog scale to measure fatigue, also showed improvement from amantadine independent of any psychiatric effects or changes in other signs or symptoms [8]. Similar results were found in subsequent careful trials using different methodologies and different outcome measures, confirming its efficacy [16,19,20].

The reason for improvement with amantadine is not known. Its original use in MS was as an antiviral agent to prevent penetration of influenza virus into the host cell, and so mitigate the severity of infection. It does not change antibodies or provoke other immune responses. There have been trials of amantadine as a therapy for MS itself, on the speculation that the disease could arise from some viral agent. In the best such study, amantadine produced fewer relapses among MS patients but no overall change in disability [21]. The study could not determine whether the drug had any direct effect on MS, and hence on MS fatigue.

Amantadine has other effects on the central nervous system, however, especially causing alterations in neurotransmitters. For example, it is useful as therapy for Parkinson's disease because it increases dopamine activity. Patients with MS who respond to amantadine show elevated levels of dopamine, as well as norepinephrine and pyruvate, and decreased lactate levels [16,22]. Vasopressin and cortisol are not affected by the drug [22]. Those patients whose fatigue responds to amantadine also show elevated levels of β-endorphin-β-lipotropin, suggesting that neuropeptides could play a role in fatigue [22]. The stimulation of opioid receptors and increased opioid release could certainly lead to a feeling of well-being and decrease in fatigue. In fact, amantadine has some value in the treatment of cocaine withdrawal. This opiate effect, if true, suggests that amantadine's antifatigue powers would not be specific for MS. That is indeed the case, since it has been shown to be useful for the fatigue of postpolio syndrome as well [23].

Amantadine may cause mild generalized central nervous system stimulation; some authors speculate that its effect is simply that of a stimulant [1]. Amantadine has also alleviated depression in isolated reports [8].

The effective dose is usually 100 mg twice daily—higher doses do not increase benefits. Side effects of amantadine that limit its usefulness include hyperactivity, insomnia, early morning awakening, hallucinations, and gastrointestinal upset. When amantadine works, the response to the drug generally occurs within 24 hours, but the fatigue returns within 24 hours after stopping the medication [6]. Overall, some two thirds of patients respond, and the benefits persist for approximately six months—but seldom longer.

Other Medications

Pemoline (Cylert) is a mild central nervous system stimulant occasionally employed in the treatment of attention deficit disorder in hyperactive children. A small but careful study demonstrated its usefulness in MS, starting at a dosage of 18.75 mg per day and increasing to 150 to 200 mg daily [10]. It is usually given as a single morning dose to minimize the side effect of insomnia.

The other drug found useful in controlled studies is clonazepam (Klonopin), given at night. At a dosage of 0.5 mg or more in the evening, patients may report less fatigue the following day. The mechanism is unclear, but because clonazepam is often sedating, the improvement in fatigue could simply result from better sleep the prior evening [24].

A number of drugs potentially useful for fatigue have proved not to be of benefit, including methylphenidate (Ritalin), pyridostigmine, steroids, and baclofen [6].

Other Therapies

Fatigue can often be managed successfully without the use of drugs. For example, management should include affirmation to the patient that fatigue is a legitimate symptom of MS; reassurance and counseling thus play a role. Other common-sense measures include rest and restructuring of daily activities (Table 11-2). Because fatigue is usually worse in

Table 11-2. Strategies found useful by MS patients for alleviating fatigue

Rest	79%
Meditation and prayer	66%
Prescription drugs	62%
Cooling the skin with water	59%
Moderate exercise	57%
Nonprescription drugs	45%
Coffee	42%

Source: Adapted from Freal et al. [2].

the afternoon, shopping, housework, and other errands should be performed in the morning.

Because MS fatigue worsens so easily with heat, measures to lower body temperature often succeed. This can be accomplished with air-conditioning, cooling baths, ice caps, and similar cooling devices. Also, aspirin effectively lowers body temperature, even in afebrile individuals, so taking two aspirin in late afternoon or before engaging in strenuous activities often helps.

Therapy and training to economize physical effort are also helpful, and energy conservation techniques are among the best treatments for fatigue [25,26]. Even though physical activity tends to worsen fatigue, moderate exercise, including formal physical therapy and conditioning, alleviates fatigue in more than half of all patients [2].

REFERENCES

1. Rolak, L. A. Multiple sclerosis. *Curr. Neurol.* 9:109, 1989.
2. Freal, J. E., Kraft, G. H., and Coryell, J. K. Symptomatic fatigue in multiple sclerosis. *Arch. Phys. Med. Rehabil.* 65:135, 1984.
3. Krupp, L. B., Alvarez, L. A., LaRocca, N. G., and Scheinberg, L. C. Fatigue in multiple sclerosis. *Arch. Neurol.* 45:435, 1988.
4. Monks, J. Experiencing symptoms in chronic illness: Fatigue in multiple sclerosis. *Int. Disabil. Studies* 11:78, 1989.
5. Jones, M. B. Long-term care insurance for people with multiple sclerosis. New York: National Multiple Sclerosis Society, Health Services Research Report, 1991.
6. Murray, T. J. Amantadine therapy for fatigue in multiple sclerosis. *Can. J. Neurol. Sci.* 12:251, 1985.
7. Burnfield, A., and Burnfield, P. Common psychological problems in multiple sclerosis. *Br. Med. J.* 1:1193, 1978.
8. Canadian MS Research Group. A randomized controlled trial of amantadine in fatigue associated with multiple sclerosis. *Can. J. Neurol. Sci.* 14:273, 1987.
9. Lawson, A., Robinson, I., and Bakes, C. Problems in evaluating the consequences of disabling illness: The case of multiple sclerosis. *Psychol. Med.* 15:555, 1985.
10. Giesser, B. Multiple sclerosis: Current concepts in management. *Drugs* 29:88, 1985.
11. Jennekens-Schinkel, A., Sanders, E. A. C. M., Lanser, J. B. K., and Vander

Velde, E. A. Reaction time in ambulant multiple sclerosis patients. *J. Neurol. Sci.* 85:173, 1988.

12. Olgiati, R., Burgunder, J.-M., and Mumenthaler, M. Increased energy cost of walking in multiple sclerosis: Effect of spasticity, ataxia, and weakness. *Arch. Phys. Med. Rehabil.* 69:846, 1988.

13. Miller, R. G., Green, A. T., Moussavi, R. S., et al. Excessive muscular fatigue in patients with spastic paraparesis. *Neurology* 40:1271, 1990.

14. Patten, B. M., Hart, A., and Lovelace, R. Multiple sclerosis associated with defects in neuromuscular transmission. *J. Neurol. Neurosurg. Psychiatry* 35:385, 1972.

15. Olgiati, R., Jacquet, J., and Prampero, P. E. Energy cost of walking and exertional dyspnea in multiple sclerosis. *Am. Rev. Respir. Dis.* 134:1005, 1986.

16. Appenzeller, O. The autonomic nervous system and fatigue. *Funct. Neurol.* 2:473, 1987.

17. Rosse, R. B. Fatigue in multiple sclerosis. *Arch. Neurol.* 46:841, 1989.

18. Rudick, R. A., and Barna, B. P. Serum interleukin-2 and soluble interleukin-2 receptor in patients with multiple sclerosis who are experiencing severe fatigue. *Arch. Neurol.* 47:254, 1990.

19. Cohen, R. A., and Fisher, M. The efficacy of amantadine on self-reported and neurobehavioral correlates of fatigue in MS. *Neurology* 38:380, 1988.

20. Schapiro, R. T. Symptom management in multiple sclerosis. New York: Demos, 1987. P. 23.

21. Plaut, G. S. The effectiveness of amantadine in reducing relapses in multiple sclerosis. *J. R. Soc. Med.* 80:91, 1987.

22. Rosenberg, G. A., and Appenzeller, O. Amantadine, fatigue, and multiple sclerosis. *Arch. Neurol.* 45:1104, 1988.

23. Dunn, M. G. Post-polio fatigue treated with amantadine. *Arch. Neurol.* 48:570, 1991.

24. Vincent, F. M. Effectiveness of clonazepam in reducing fatigue associated with multiple sclerosis. *Neurology* 38:380, 1988.

25. Erickson, R. P., Lie, M. R., and Wineinger, M. A. Rehabilitation in multiple sclerosis. *Mayo Clin. Proc.* 64:818, 1989.

26. Krupp, L. B., LaRocca, N. G., Muir-Nash, J., and Steinberg, A. D. The fatigue severity scale: Application to patients with multiple sclerosis and systemic lupus erythematosus. *Arch. Neurol.* 46:1121, 1989.

12

Louis Reik, Jr.

Lyme Disease and Fatigue

Lyme disease is a widely distributed, multisystem infection caused by a tick-transmitted spirochete, *Borrelia burgdorferi*. The disease has been reported from five continents: Africa, Asia, Australia, Europe, and North America, where it occurs both in Canada and in the United States [1–3]. Within the United States, Lyme disease is the most common tick-transmitted illness, and it has been acquired there in 43 states. It is endemic in the upper Midwest and in coastal mid-Atlantic and southern New England states; it is most common in New York, New Jersey, Pennsylvania, Connecticut, Massachusetts, Rhode Island, Wisconsin, and Minnesota [3].

The usual vectors are several small, hard-bodied ticks of the genus *Ixodes* [4,5]. In North America, the main vector in the Northeast and Midwest is *I. dammini*, the deer tick. *I. pacificus*, the western black-legged tick, is the most important vector on the West Coast.

Ixodes species have a three-stage life cycle (larva, nymph, adult) [4,5]. The larval ticks are infected by feeding on reservoir hosts (various birds and small mammals). Following feeding, infection is maintained through successive molts to the nymphal and adult stages. Consequently, the bite of either can result in Lyme disease.

But transmission generally takes some time. Infection after less than 24 hours of attachment is rare [6], and transmission can be prevented in many cases if the tick is removed as soon as possible. Removal is best accomplished by grasping the tick with fine tweezers as close to the skin

161

as possible and pulling gently [7]. Other methods are riskier: squeezing or twisting the tick can cause regurgitation of gut contents and increase the chance of infection.

In the case of *I dammini*, the most important North American vector, it is the smaller (2 mm) nymph that most often bites humans. Since the nymphs feed most actively from May to July, North American Lyme disease begins most often in summer.

GENERAL CLINICAL FEATURES

Both humans and animals are affected. Infected dogs, cows, and horses develop arthritis. Infected cows have also had mastitis, spontaneous abortion, myocarditis, nephritis, and pneumonitis, while infected horses have had swelling of the legs, weight loss, dermatitis, conjunctivitis, panuveitis, nasal discharge, and cough. Encephalitis in horses and facial palsy and meningitis in dogs have also been linked to *B. burgdorferi* infection [2].

In humans, the skin, heart, nervous system, and joints are the organ systems most often involved, frequently in stages [1,8]. Early infection (stage 1) begins with the localized skin lesion, erythema migrans (EM). Dissemination (stage 2) follows within days to weeks and may be followed in turn, weeks to months later, by intermittent symptoms that lead finally to late or persistent infection (stage 3) beginning a year or more after the onset of infection. In an individual patient, any or all stages may be present.

Early Localized Infection (Stage 1)

The illness usually begins 3 days to 1 month after an infective tick bite, with a red papule or macule that starts at the site of the bite and expands centrifugally as *B. burgdorferi* proliferates and spreads locally in the skin [1,8–11]. As the lesion expands, it clears centrally to form an annular erythema, EM, the best clinical marker for early disease (present in 80% of North American patients). Accompanying regional adenopathy is common (40% of cases), but severe constitutional symptoms are not. Typically, the erythema fades and disappears within 3 or 4 weeks, even without treatment.

Early Disseminated Infection (Stage 2)

Within days to weeks after inoculation, *B. burgdorferi* can spread hematogenously to other skin sites and to the heart, nervous system, muscle, eye, bone, joints, and reticuloendothelial system.

Skin

Multiple secondary skin lesions, similar to but smaller and less migratory than the initial EM, develop in about 25% of North American patients [1,10]. Systemic symptoms are more intense then, and there may be signs reflecting spread of infection to the other organ systems. Eventually, within weeks to months after illness onset, B. burgdorferi appears to settle and become sequestered in certain of these tissues

Localization in the skin causes lymphocytoma cutis or borrelial lymphocytoma cutis, a nodular solitary red or purple lesion containing lymphoid follicles and ranging from a few millimeters to several centimeters in size [8]. Most common on the nipple in adults and on the earlobe in children, lymphocytoma can develop for as long as 6 to 10 months after a tick bite and persist for years without treatment.

Nervous System

Localization in the nervous system can produce symptoms while EM is still present, but it does so more often 1 to 6 months after the skin lesion has faded. Fifteen to 20% of North American patients are affected. The most common neurologic abnormalities are lymphocytic meningitis, radicular pains, and cranial and peripheral neuropathies, sometimes accompanied by central nervous system (CNS) parenchymal signs and symptoms [1,2,9,12,13].

Eighty percent have meningitis, the symptoms recurring in attacks several weeks long alternating with similar periods of milder symptoms over 1 to many months in untreated cases [2,12,13]. Lymphocytic pleocytosis is typical (100–200 cells/µl), and the cerebrospinal fluid (CSF) contains excess protein, increased levels of immunoglobulins G and M (IgG and IgM), oligoclonal bands of IgG, and locally synthesized anti-B. burgdorferi antibody [2,12,13].

Nearly half of the patients have CNS symptoms in addition [2,12,13]. The symptoms are usually mild and fluctuate like the meningeal symptoms, either in concert with them or independently. Most common are somnolence, emotional lability, depression, impaired memory and concentration, and behavioral change. Occasional patients develop more severe CNS abnormalities including chorea, cerebellar ataxia, seizures, dementia, hemiplegia, transverse myelitis, focal or multifocal encephalitis, and leukoencephalitis [2,12].

The peripheral neuropathy is usually asymmetric, mixed sensorimotor, multifocal, and axonal. Typical patterns include mononeuritis simplex and multiplex, motor or sensory radiculitis on the trunk or extremities, and asymmetric radiculoplexitis. The most common cranial neuropathy is facial palsy: as many as 10% of North American patients with Lyme disease may develop it, and it is bilateral in up to one-third of cases. Any of the cranial nerves may be involved, however, sometimes in multiples [2,12,13].

All of these neurologic abnormalities usually subside, even without treatment, but severe CNS abnormalities often resolve only partially and residual disability is common.

Heart

Localization in the heart also produces symptoms within weeks of illness onset. About 4% of North American patients are affected, and symptoms last for days to 6 weeks. Fluctuating atrioventricular block is most common. Heart block can progress to asystole and require a temporary pacemaker, but usually for no more than a week. Diffuse myocarditis, left ventricular dysfunction, pericarditis, and fatal pancarditis can also occur, but less often [1,14].

Joints

Eighty percent of untreated North American patients with Lyme disease develop joint involvement [1,9,10,15]. One-fourth of them experience attacks of migratory joint, periarticular, or musculoskeletal pain without ever developing objective joint abnormalities [1,15]. The pain usually begins 2 weeks (range, 1 day to 8 weeks) after the skin lesion first appears and lasts for hours to days in any one location. It typically affects one or two sites at a time, and can migrate to as many as 10 sites in all during a single attack. Later in the course of the disease, the pain settles in just one or a few joints where it recurs for months to years (mean, 3 years) in attacks lasting a few days followed by months of remission [1,15].

In another half of the untreated cases, objective joint abnormalities do develop [1,15]. Attacks of frank arthritis begin 4 days to 2 years after illness onset (mean, 6 months), often following earlier episodes of migratory arthralgia (50% of cases) [1,15]. Individual patients may experience as few as one or as many as 12 episodes of arthritis lasting 3 days to 11.5 months (mean, 3 months) and recurring over 1 to 8 years before resolving [1,15,16].

Late Infection (Stage 3)

Joints

In most cases, the attacks of arthritis become less severe, less frequent, and of shorter duration with time, and the number of patients with recurrences decreases by 10 to 20% yearly. But in 10% of cases, the attacks last progressively longer until chronic arthritis (defined as lasting continuously for a year or more) eventually ensues, usually about a year after illness onset (range, 4 months to 4 years). One to three joints are typically involved, most often the knee, hip, or shoulder. Erosion of cartilage and bone and permanent disability can result. But even this chronic arthritis generally improves over time without treatment: continuous joint inflammation for more than several years is rare [1,15,16].

Skin

Persistent skin infection causes acrodermatitis chronica atrophicans (ACA) [8]. ACA is a chronic disorder that begins gradually 6 months to 10 years after illness onset and progresses slowly: it does not remit spontaneously. It begins asymmetrically, usually on the distal extremities, with bluish-red discoloration and doughy swelling of the skin that can persist for years or even decades. Eventually, the inflammation is replaced by atrophy of the skin and underlying tissues. Accompanying signs and symptoms include polyneuropathy, local joint deformity, fatigue, weight loss, and personality change.

Nervous System

Persisting *B. burgdorferi* infection also causes both central and peripheral nervous system abnormalities. The best defined is progressive borrelia encephalomyelitis, a disorder reported mainly from Europe but occurring also in North America [2,17]. Progressive encephalomyelitis can follow EM or meningopolyneuritis by as long as 7 years; it occasionally appears earlier, within months of illness onset. Systemic signs and symptoms are usually absent. Once it does begin, it follows either a progressive or remitting relapsing course; like ACA, it does not resolve spontaneously. Nervous system involvement is diffuse and multifocal, and the abnormalities seen include encephalopathy (diffuse, multifocal, or both), seizures, dementia, hemiplegia, dysphasia, hemianopia, paraparesis and quadriparesis, cranial nerve palsies, and radiculoneuropathy.

The CSF is typically abnormal and contains excess lymphocytes (up to 2300 μl; usually 100–200), increased protein (up to 1800 mg/dl), and locally synthesized IgG and specific anti-*B. burgdorferi* antibody. Computerized tomography (CT) and magnetic resonance imaging (MRI) have shown infarct patterns, multifocal white matter abnormalities in the hemispheres and brainstem, and hydrocephalus. Cerebral angiography has shown changes consistent with vasculitis [2,17].

Progressive borrelia encephalomyelitis is rare among North American patients with Lyme disease, but less striking CNS abnormalities are frequent [2, 18–20]. Affected patients have defects in memory, concentration, and mood. All ages are affected, the symptoms beginning months to years after the beginning of infection and persisting for years if not treated. In the worst cases, bedside tests of mental function are abnormal. In milder cases, abnormalities may be apparent only on more detailed neuropsychologic testing.

There are usually no physical signs of CNS dysfunction, although accompanying signs of polyneuropathy are common [2,18–20]. The CSF protein is elevated in one-third or more of patients [18], and locally synthesized specific antibody is present in 40 to 70% [18–20]; but pleocytosis is only occasionally present, and IgG abnormalities are seldom detected [2,18–20]. Electroencephalograms and CT are usually normal, but MRI shows multiple punctate areas of increased signal in the cerebral white matter in 15 to 40% of those affected [18–20].

A mild multifocal polyneuropathy is also common among North American patients with late Lyme disease, as many as 50% of whom may have distal, asymmetric, intermittent limb paresthesias [18,19,21]. These begin months after illness onset and usually have been present for a year or more by the time of diagnosis. Twenty-five percent also have radicular pains, especially in the legs, and a similar number have the carpal tunnel syndrome [22]. Physical findings are usually confined to a mild, stocking-and-glove pattern, distal sensory loss without motor weakness or reflex change. Electrophysiologic testing shows multifocal, mainly distal, axonal abnormalities in 40 to 50% of patients with late disease [18,19,21]. As many as 70% of those affected may have an increase in CSF protein content, or intrathecal concentration of specific antibody, or both [18]. Pleocytosis is unusual.

In Europe, where ACA is more common, 25 to 70% of patients with this and other late sclerotic skin lesions also have peripheral neuropathy [2,8,23]. Although symptoms are often more intense and physical findings more common than in North American patients with neuropathy and stage 3 disease, the electrophysiologic abnormalities are the same.

FATIGUE IN LYME DISEASE

Early Disease

Constitutional symptoms, including fatigue, are typically mild and transient in early localized disease (stage 1) [1,10]. They become more prominent later when *B. burgdorferi* spreads hematogenously to cause disseminated disease (stage 2). Then systemic symptoms intensify and fatigue is common (30 to 80% of patients with EM) [1,9,10,24,25]. Fatigue seldom occurs alone, however. It is usually accompanied by other systemic symptoms including fever, chills, malaise, lethargy, headache, neck stiffness, musculoskeletal and joint pains, cough, and sore throat. Accompanying signs, other than EM, may include generalized adenopathy, splenomegaly, malar rash, periorbital edema, and conjunctivitis. But only the lethargy and fatigue tend to be constant, forming a persistent background of illness on which the other symptoms, intermittent and changing, are periodically superimposed [1,8,10,26]. Occasionally, fatigue precedes EM or, in those cases in which EM never develops (20 to 40% of North American patients), occurs without it [1,8]. Then influenza or infectious mononucleosis can be simulated.

These symptoms of early disseminated infection typically subside within weeks or a month or two, even without treatment. But fatigue can persist for months after the skin lesion and its associated symptoms have faded, and frequently is still present when symptoms of later organ system involvement appear [10]. Fatigue is common in patients with cardiac involvement. It also affects as many as 65% of patients with early neurologic disease, especially those with meningitis, and fluctuates in intensity along with their headache, neck stiffness, nausea, vomiting, and malaise [2,12,27].

Fatigue is frequent too among patients who develop joint involvement. It is common early in the course in those with migratory arthralgias, and can persist for months in between the attacks of joint pain [1,9,10,15]. Later on, fatigue is less persistent, but it recurs during the attacks in 40% of cases [15]. Fatigue also accompanies arthritic attacks in 30 to 40% of patients who develop acute arthritis and can recur periodically in between the attacks in about the same number, either alone or accompanied by periarticular or joint pain [1,15]. Other systemic signs and symptoms are less common but include fever, headache, neck stiffness, abdominal pain, recurrent EM, and regional or generalized lymphadenopathy [1,9,10,15].

Late Disease

Among patients with chronic arthritis, fatigue is common (70% of patients), frequently intense, and often persistent [1,15]. Additional signs and symptoms are unusual aside from occasional myalgia (20%) or regional lymphadenopathy (20%).

Persistent and profound fatigue can accompany other manifestations of late Lyme disease as well. While fatigue is infrequent in patients with ACA, it does occur in 6% [8].

Patients with late neurologic involvement are affected more commonly, the fatigue typically beginning along with the neurologic complaints months to years after the onset of infection and, like the neurologic complaints, persisting for years if not treated. In one study, fatigue was a prominent symptom in 20 of 27 patients with late Lyme disease and polyneuropathy, encephalopathy, or both [18]. Associated complaints included headache in 13 patients and arthritis in 10, in addition to the usual neurologic symptoms (paresthesias, radicular pains, memory loss, difficulty concentrating, and mood changes).

The causes of and interrelationships among the disabilities of late neurologic disease are not clear, however. Lyme disease patients with encephalopathy typically have memory defects on neuropsychologic tests [18,19,28,29], and as many as 30% have evidence of depression on the Minnesota Multiphasic Personality Inventory test [29]. As compared to normal controls, patients do have high fatigue and depression scores and defects in recall, long-term retrieval, and long-term memory storage [30]. But they do not differ significantly in these neuropsychologic measures from patients with chronic fatigue alone or from patients recovered from Lyme disease who still complain of fatigue and cognitive difficulties but have no objective findings [30]. It seems possible that at least some of their complaints may originate in or be influenced by depression or stress [29,30].

Indeed, in a number of cases, chronic fatigue in Lyme disease has been linked to fibromyalgia rather than to active infection. Both Dinerman and Steere [31] and Sigal [32] have described patients who developed persistent fatigue, chronic headache, generalized aching and stiffness, and multiple tender points in relation to Lyme disease. The symptoms began along with or soon after those of early Lyme disease, or months to years (up to 4 years) later along with symptoms of late disease (encephalopathy, neuropathy, or chronic arthritis). The symptoms were long lasting and had been present a mean of 10.5 months in one study and 4.1 years in the other. In both studies, the signs of active Lyme disease resolved following antibiotic therapy while the symptoms of fibromyalgia did not, suggesting that active *B. burgdorferi* infection was required to trigger the syndrome but not for its persistence. The triggering factor may be CNS involvement. Dinerman and Steere [31] observed that fibromyalgia developed primarily in patients with neurologic abnormalities, and Sigal [32] suggested that CNS involvement first caused a sleep disorder that ultimately precipitated the musculoskeletal symptoms.

The frequency of *B. burgdorferi* infection among unselected patients presenting with fibromyalgia has not been studied, but it is probably not high. In one study of 60 English patients with the related syndrome of myalgic encephalomyelitis (postviral fatigue), only six had positive serum antibody tests and none of these had positive immunoblots [33].

To my knowledge, the frequency of *B. burgdorferi* infection among unselected patients presenting with chronic fatigue has not been studied either. Nor is it certain how often chronic fatigue occurs as the solitary late manifestation in patients already known to have Lyme disease.

It probably seldom does so, however. Szer et al. [16] followed 46 children with untreated early Lyme disease prospectively for 10 to 13 years and described only one with persisting fatigue as his sole symptom; the patient refused further evaluation so the presence of other abnormalities could not be assessed. From their extensive experience with Lyme disease, Pachner and Steere [34] described just four other patients with severe, incapacitating fatigue late in the illness, which they attributed to nervous system involvement. In two of them the fatigue was episodic, occurring in repeated attacks lasting days to weeks. One patient had a Babinski sign and the other three were said to be normal neurologically. But they did not report how often accompanying arthritis was present. Moreover, in the absence of neuropsychologic testing, it is uncertain that encephalopathy was not present in addition.

DIAGNOSIS OF FATIGUE CAUSED BY LYME DISEASE

Laboratory Diagnosis

The laboratory diagnosis of fatigue from Lyme disease is usually made indirectly, by demonstrating an immune response to *B. burgdorferi*, rather than directly: Isolation of the spirochete from patients is difficult, and the small number of organisms present prevents their routine identification in stained sections of infected tissues.

When fatigue is the result of early disease, nonspecific laboratory abnormalities can provide a diagnostic lead—the erythrocyte sedimentation rate is often elevated, serum levels of IgM may be increased, and the serum may contain cryoimmunoglobulins and other circulating immune complexes [1,8–11]. But other routine laboratory tests are usually normal; and, in patients whose fatigue is caused by late disease, even these few abnormalities are typically absent.

The serum of most patients with fatigue caused by disseminated Lyme disease does contain specific anti-*B. burgdorferi* antibodies, however, and detection of their presence is the best laboratory proof of the illness [1,35–38]. These antibodies can be measured by either indirect immunofluorescent (IFA) or enzyme-linked immunosorbent assay (ELISA). In most laboratories, the more sensitive and more specific ELISA technique is used, and IgG and IgM antibodies are measured separately.

Specific IgM antibodies appear first, 2 to 4 weeks after the start of infection [1,35–38]. Their levels peak at 6 to 8 weeks and then decline. Raised levels of IgM antibodies can persist throughout the course of the infection in occasional cases, however. IgG antibodies appear later, the titers becoming elevated during the second and third months of infection [1,35–38]. Once elevated IgG titers can remain high for years, even after successful antibiotic treatment or during spontaneous remission.

Hence, high titers of serum IgM anti-*B. burgdorferi* antibody indicate acute infection, whereas high titers of IgG antibody can indicate either active or past infection. Patients with EM alone either are seronegative or have high serum titers of IgM antibody, while those with early disseminated disease and fatigue typically have raised levels of either IgG antibodies alone or both IgG and IgM antibodies. Patients with fatigue due to late disease almost always have elevated levels of IgG antibodies alone [1,35–38].

Yet the diagnosis of fatigue due to Lyme disease should be made clinically in any case, and only confirmed serologically. Indeed, caution is necessary when interpreting individual antibody test results from patients with fatigue who are suspected of having Lyme disease. These tests are not standardized, and there is considerable variability within and between laboratories [39–41]. Moreover, false-positive tests can occur in patients with other spirochetal diseases, rheumatoid arthritis, bacterial endocarditis, infectious mononucleosis, Rocky Mountain spotted fever, and tuberculous meningitis [42,43]. Most often, false-positive tests result from low titers of cross-reacting IgM antibodies, but patients with syphilis or relapsing fever can have high titers of cross-reacting IgG antibodies [42].

Such false-positive results can be identified through the serum immunoblot [44,45]. This test is more sensitive than the ELISA, and it is sometimes positive earlier in the illness. Furthermore, the immunoblot is more specific than the ELISA, as long as a sufficient number of antibody bands is required for a positive result. Many normal individuals have antibodies against one or more B. burgdorferi antigens, as do some patients with rheumatic diseases, syphilis, or relapsing fever [37]; but most patients with Lyme disease can be distinguished from these others because they have antibodies reacting with many more antigens [44].

Still, no serologic measure—regardless of titer—accurately reflects disease activity, and the presence of serum immunity by itself is not sufficient to diagnose fatigue caused by active Lyme disease. Even a truly positive test result may indicate only past exposure to B. burgdorferi rather than active infection with it [2,46,47]. From 8 to 23% of residents in hyperendemic areas, and 15 to 25% of those with recreational or vocational outdoor exposure, have positive tests for anti-B. burgdorferi antibody by IFA or ELISA. Because the ratio of seropositivity from simple exposure to positivity from symptomatic infection has been 1 : 1 in several serologic surveys [46,47], the predictive value of a positive serum antibody test is likely to be low.

Furthermore, high titers of specific serum antibodies are not always present in patients with fatigue from active Lyme disease. In some cases, the level of serum IgM antibody is not raised when EM debuts [35–38] and may not be so even when early neurologic involvement begins weeks later [2,48]. In others, early treatment with oral antibiotics abrogates the humoral immune response without fully eradicating the organism, especially from the CNS. Then late nervous system involvement with its attendant fatigue can arise in a seronegative patient [2,37,49]. Because seronegativity may be only apparent—specific antibody may be present in CSF [48], serum immunoblots may be positive [44], or specific antibody may be sequestered in immune complexes in serum or CSF [50]—in some cases the diagnosis will have to be made and treatment prescribed on clinical grounds alone.

Clinical Diagnosis

Patients with fatigue caused by active B. burgdorferi infection almost always have other signs and symptoms of the illness. Although fatigue may persist while other symptoms come and go, it seldom if ever occurs alone as the sole manifestation of Lyme disease. In cases of early disseminated disease, clinical features indicating that fatigue is due to Lyme disease include EM, typical constitutional symptoms, and accompanying signs and symptoms of involvement of the nervous system, heart, re-ticuloendothelial system, or joints. Epidemiologic clues to early disease are only suggestive, but they include a history of tick bite, onset in summer, and travel or residence in an endemic area. In cases of late Lyme disease, the accompanying clinical features that indicate fatigue is due to active *B. burgdorferi* infection are ACA, chronic arthritis, en-cephalopathy, and neuropathy. Fibromyalgia by itself does not signify active Lyme disease; and randomly selected patients with chronic fatigue alone, without previous objective findings of Lyme disease, are not likely to have active Lyme disease as a cause of their symptoms.

Consequently, the definite diagnosis of fatigue caused by active Lyme disease requires the presence of fatigue without other cause plus serum or CSF reactivity against *B. burgdorferi* and at least one of the following: (1) well-documented EM, (3) lymphocytoma, (3) ACA, (4) other organ system involvement typical of Lyme disease (heart, joints, or nervous system), or (5) seroconversion or fourfold rise in titer of paired serum specimens. Lyme disease can still be suspected and treated if these criteria are not all satisfied, but the diagnosis is then uncertain and other possibilities should be considered first.

TREATMENT AND RESPONSE

B. burgdorferi is sensitive in vitro to a variety of commonly used antibiotics [1,2]. It is most sensitive to ceftriaxone, cefotaxime, and erythromycin; less so to the tetracyclines, amoxicillin, imipenem, lincomycin, chlor-amphenicol, and ciprofloxacin; and only moderately sensitive to peni-cillin. It is resistant to ofloxacin, the aminoglycosides, rifampin, and trimethoprim. The antibiotic sensitivities of *B. burgdorferi* measured in vivo in experimentally infected laboratory animals generally parallel those measured in vitro, except that erythromycin is not as effective [1,2].

Which of these antibiotics is best for treating human Lyme disease is not certain, however, and the most effective regimens probably remain to be defined. At present, early disease (localized stage 1 or disseminated stage 2) is usually treated with oral doxycycline or amoxicillin (Table 12-1) [1,2,51]. Amoxicillin is also the drug of choice for children with early disease, but erythromycin is substituted for those with penicillin allergy. The duration of treatment with each of these antibiotics is typ-ically 10 to 30 days, depending on the severity of the initial symptoms and the clinical response. Patients with more severe early disease (mul-tiple EM or EM with constitutional symptoms) respond less quickly to treatment. Occasionally, retreatment is necessary [1,2,51].

When oral antibiotics are prescribed for early Lyme disease, signs and symptoms usually improve within 3 weeks [24,52] but they may worsen initially. The symptoms of 10 to 15% of patients intensify temporarily after the first dose or two (Jarisch-Herxheimer reaction), often accom-

Table 12-1. Antibiotic therapy for Lyme disease

Manifestation	Treatment[a]
Early Infection	
LOCALIZED (STAGE 1)	
Adults	Doxycycline, 100 mg po BID × 10–30 days
	Amoxicillin, 500 mg po QID × 10–30 days[b]
Children (≤ 8 yr)	Amoxicillin, 20–40 mg/kg/day in 4 divided doses × 10–30 days
	Erythromycin, 30 mg/kg/day in 4 divided doses × 10–30 days in cases of penicillin allergy
DISSEMINATED (STAGE 2)	
Facial palsy	Oral antibiotics as for stage 1
Other neurologic	
Adults	Penicillin G, 20–24 million units/day IV × 10–14 days
	Ceftriaxone, 2 g/day × 2–4 wk
	Doxycycline, 100–200 mg po BID × 10–30 days
Children	Penicillin G, 250,000 units/kg/day IV in divided doses q4h × 10–14 days
	Ceftriaxone, 50–80 mg/kg/day IV × 2–4 wk
Cardiac	
First-degree A-V block	Oral antibiotics as for stage 1
High degree block	IV penicillin or ceftriaxone as for neurologic involvement
Acute arthritis	Doxycycline, 100 mg po BID × 30 days
	Amoxicillin, 500 mg, plus probenecid, 500 mg po qid × 30 days
	Ceftriaxone, 2 g/day IV × 14 days
	Penicillin G, 20 million units/day × 14 days
Late Infection (Stage 3)	
Acrodermatitis	Stage 1 oral regimens for 30 days
Neurologic involvement	IV penicillin or ceftriaxone or oral doxycycline as for stage 2 neurologic involvement
Chronic arthritis	As for stage 2 acute arthritis

[a]Duration of treatment depends on the clinical response.
[b]May be combined with probenecid 500 mg po qid.

panied by profound fatigue [1,2,24,51]. The reaction settles quickly and requires no special treatment. More delayed reactions to therapy can develop too: symptoms intensify between the second and twentieth days of treatment in another 5 to 10% of cases [24]. Fatigue is again common and sometimes profound, but this reaction also requires no special treatment, and it typically resolves within 3 weeks.

Other patients with early Lyme disease may continue to have symptoms or experience late complications in spite of antibiotic therapy. How often symptoms persist following treatment depends at least partly on the antibiotics prescribed. Following early treatment protocols using penicillin, tetracycline, or erythromycin, nearly half of the patients continued to have minor symptoms (recurrent headaches, arthralgias, musculoskeletal pain, lethargy, fatigue), sometimes for years [1]. Yet in a more recent series of EM patients treated orally for 21 days with either doxycycline or amoxicillin and probenecid, 85% were symptom free when evaluated 3 months later. Among the others who continued to have symptoms, 7% experienced arthralgias, 4% fatigue, and 4% both [53].

Severity of initial illness is another factor in the persistence of symptoms after treatment. Residual symptoms are more common among treated patients who have had multiple EMs or EM with constitutional symptoms [52,54,55]. However, it is not clear whether these persisting symptoms result from continuing infection or are parainfectious instead. Clinical observations suggest the latter: They seldom respond to repeated courses of antibiotics, and they do tend to disappear with time.

For some patients with early disseminated disease, oral antibiotic therapy may not be enough. Antibiotics are usually given intravenously to patients with nervous system abnormalities (except for isolated facial palsy) and to those with severe cardiac involvement [1,2,51]. High-dose penicillin and ceftriaxone are both effective, although ceftriaxone is often favored in neurologic cases because of its better penetration into the CSF. Doxycycline can be substituted when there is penicillin allergy.

When patients with neurologic complaints are treated parenterally, both the meningeal and constitutional symptoms generally improve within days. CSF cell counts are usually lower by the end of therapy, but parenchymal neurologic signs resolve more slowly and sometimes incompletely [1,2,56]. Residual symptoms (fatigue, arthralgias, musculoskeletal pain) can still occur in spite of intravenous antibiotic therapy [2,56]; but, like the similar symptoms that persist following oral treatment, they seldom respond to repeated courses of antibiotics.

Among patients with late (stage 3) Lyme disease, oral antibiotic therapy usually cures those with ACA [1,8]. Late nervous system disease is normally treated parenterally, however. Progressive encephalomyelitis responds promptly to intravenous penicillin or ceftriaxone with disappearance of pleocytosis and a halt in the progression of disability, although residual neurologic abnormalities are common [2,17]. For patients with late encephalopathy or polyneuropathy, intravenous ceftriaxone is most effective [2,57]. But there is little improvement during the course of treatment itself, and recovery afterward is slow: Some improvement may be evident 2 months later, while maximum recovery may take 6 months. The treatment of Lyme arthritis is less satisfactory. Arthritis often does not respond to antibiotic treatment, failing just as frequently after either oral or parenteral therapy [1].

If symptoms improve following treatment but then recur (recrudescent symptoms), retreatment for a longer course is indicated. When symptoms, particularly if they are nonspecific, persist following treatment (residual symptoms), repeated courses of antibiotic therapy typically are not effective. Fibromyalgia does not respond to antibiotic therapy and is best treated with antidepressants and a graded exercise program [31,32]. Isolated fatigue, without other symptoms of active Lyme disease, is unlikely to respond to antibiotics either. Seropositive patients with chronic fatigue who have not previously been treated with parenteral antibiotics should be given a single 1-month course, preferably of ceftriaxone. If there is no response to treatment, further antibiotic therapy is not indicated.

CONCLUSION

Antibiotic treatment in patients with Lyme disease and fatigue should be directed at more objective signs of active disease and not at the fatigue. In most cases, the fatigue will improve along with the other signs and symptoms, albeit more slowly. If it does not, additional courses of antibiotics will not help.

REFERENCES

1. Steere, A.C. Lyme disease. *N. Engl. J. Med.* 321:586, 1989.
2. Reik, L. *Lyme Disease and the Nervous System.* New York: Thieme Medical Publishers, 1991.
3. Centers for Disease Control. Lyme disease—United States, 1987 and 1988. *M.M.W.R.* 38:668, 1989.
4. Burgdorfer, W. Vector/host relationships of the Lyme disease spirochete, *Borrelia burgdorferi. Rheum. Dis. Clin. North Am.* 15:775, 1989.
5. Anderson, J.F. Epizootiology of *Borrelia* in *Ixodes* tick vectors and reservoir hosts. *Rev. Infect. Dis.* 11 (Suppl. 6):S1451, 1989.
6. Piesman, J., Mather, T.N., Sinsky, R.J., and Spielman, A. Duration of tick attachment and *Borrelia burgdorferi* transmission. *J. Clin. Microbiol.* 25:557, 1987.
7. Anderson, J.F. Preventing Lyme disease. *Rheum. Dis. Clin. North Am.* 15:757, 1989.
8. Åsbrink, E., and Hovmark, A. Early and late cutaneous manifestations in *Ixodes*-borne borreliosis (erythema migrans borreliosis, Lyme borreliosis). *Ann. N.Y. Acad. Sci.* 539:4, 1988.
9. Steere, A.C., Malawista, S.E., Hardin, J.A., et al. Erythema chronicum migrans and Lyme arthritis: The enlarging clinical spectrum. *Ann. Intern. Med.* 86:685, 1977.
10. Steere, A.C., Bartenhagen, N.H., Craft, J.E., et al. The early clinical manifestations of Lyme disease. *Ann. Intern. Med.* 99:76, 1983.
11. Shrestha, M., Grodzicki, R.L., and Steere, A.C. Diagnosing early Lyme disease. *Am. J. Med.* 78:235, 1985.
12. Reik, L., Steere, A.C., Bartenhagen, N.H., et al. Neurologic abnormalities of Lyme disease. *Medicine* 58:281, 1979.

13. Pachner, A.R., and Steere, A.C. The triad of neurologic manifestations of Lyme disease: Meningitis, cranial neuritis and radiculoneuritis. *Neurology* 35:47, 1985.
14. Steere, A.C., Batsford, W.P., Weinberg, M., et al. Lyme carditis: Cardiac abnormalities of Lyme disease. *Ann. Intern. Med.* 93:8, 1980.
15. Steere, A.C., Schoen, R.T., and Taylor, E. The clinical evolution of Lyme arthritis. *Ann. Intern. Med.* 107:725, 1987.
16. Szer, I.S., Taylor, E., and Steere, A.C. The long-term course of Lyme arthritis in children. *N. Engl. J. Med.* 325:159, 1991.
17. Ackermann, R., Rehse-Küpper, B., Gollmer, E., and Schmidt, R. Chronic neurologic manifestations of erythema migrans borreliosis. *Ann. N.Y. Acad. Sci.* 539:16, 1988.
18. Logigian, E.L., Kaplan, R.F., and Steere, A.C. Chronic neurologic manifestations of Lyme disease. *N. Engl. J. Med.* 323:1438, 1990.
19. Halperin, J.J., Pass, H.L., Anand, A.K., et al. Nervous system abnormalities in Lyme disease. *Ann. N.Y. Acad. Sci.* 539:24, 1988.
20. Halperin, J.J., Krupp, L.B., Golightly, M.G., and Volkman, D.J. Lyme-borreliosis-associated encephalopathy. *Neurology* 40:1340, 1990.
21. Halperin, J.J., Little, B.W., Coyle, P.K., and Dattwyler, R.J. Lyme disease: Cause of a treatable peripheral neuropathy. *Neurology* 37:1700, 1987.
22. Halperin, J.J., Volkman, D.J., Luft, B.J., and Dattwyler, R.J. Carpal tunnel syndrome in Lyme borreliosis. *Muscle Nerve* 12:397, 1989.
23. Kristoferitsch, W., Sluga, E., Graf, M., et al. Neuropathy associated with acrodermatitis chronica atrophicans: Clinical and morphological features. *Ann. N.Y. Acad. Sci.* 539:35, 1988.
24. Weber, K., and Neubert, U. Clinical features of early erythema migrans disease and related disorders. *Zentralbl. Bakteriol. Mikrobiol. Hyg. [A]* 236:209, 1986.
25. Åsbrink, E., Olsson, I., and Hovmark, A. Erythema chronicum migrans Afzelius in Sweden: A study on 231 patients. *Zentralbl. Bakteriol. Mikrobiol. Hyg. [A]* 236:229, 1986.
26. Steere, A.C., Bartenhagen, N.H., Craft, J.E., et al. Clinical manifestations of Lyme disease. *Zentralbl. Bakteriol. Mikrobiol. Hyg. [A]* 236:201, 1986.
27. Stiernstedt, G.T., Gustafsson, R., Karlsson, M., et al. Clinical manifestations and diagnosis of neuroborreliosis. *Ann. N.Y. Acad. Sci.* 539:46, 1988.
28. Krupp, L.B., Fernquist, S., Masur, D., and Halperin, J.J. Cognitive impairment in Lyme disease. *Neurology* 40 (Suppl. 1):304, 1990.
29. Kaplan, R.F., Vincent, L.C., Meadows, M.E., et al. Neuropsychological impairment in Lyme disease. Presented at the American Psychological Association Annual Convention, August 1990.
30. Krupp, L.B., LaRocca, N.G., Luft, B.J., and Halperin, J.J. Comparison of neurologic and psychologic findings in patients with Lyme disease and chronic fatigue syndrome. *Neurology* 39 (Suppl. 1):144, 1989.
31. Dinerman, H., and Steere, A.C. Fibromyalgia following Lyme disease: Association with neurologic involvement and lack of response to antibiotic therapy. *Arthritis Rheum.* 33:S136, 1990.
32. Sigal, L.H. Summary of the first 100 patients seen at a Lyme disease referral center. *Am. J. Med.* 88:577, 1990.
33. Wright, D.J.M., Mulhemann, D.F., Williams, D.G., and Behan, P.O. Postviral fatigue and borrelial antibodies. *Ann. N.Y. Acad. Sci.* 539:507, 1988.
34. Pachner, A.R., and Steere, A.C. CNS manifestations of third stage Lyme disease. *Zentralbl. Bakteriol. Mikrobiol. Hyg. [A]* 236:301, 1986.
35. Magnarelli, L.A. Laboratory diagnosis of Lyme disease. *Rheum. Dis. Clin. North Am.* 15:735, 1989.

36. Dattwyler, R.J., Volkman, D.J., and Luft, B.J. Immunologic aspects of Lyme borreliosis. *Rev. Infect. Dis.* 11 (Suppl. 6):S1494, 1989.
37. Magnarelli, L.A. Serologic diagnosis of Lyme disease. *Ann. N.Y. Acad. Sci.* 539:154, 1988.
38. Steere, A.C., Grodzicki, R.L., Kornblatt, A.N., et al. The spirochetal etiology of Lyme disease. *N. Engl. J. Med.* 308:740, 1983.
39. Hedberg, C.W., Osterholm, M.T., MacDonald, K.L., and White, K.E. An interlaboratory study of antibody to *Borrelia burgdorferi*. *J. Infect. Dis.* 155:1325, 1987.
40. Schwartz, B.S., Goldstein, M.D., Ribeiro, J.M.C., et al. Antibody testing in Lyme disease: A comparison of results in four laboratories. *J.A.M.A.* 262:3431, 1989.
41. Luger, S.W., and Krauss, E. Serologic tests for Lyme disease: Interlaboratory variability. *Arch. Intern. Med.* 150:761, 1990.
42. Magnarelli, L.A., Anderson, J.F., and Johnson, R.C. Cross-reactivity in serological tests for Lyme disease and other spirochetal infections. *J. Infect. Dis.* 156:183, 1987.
43. Kaell, A., Volkman, D., Gorevic, P., et al. Positive Lyme serology in subacute bacterial endocarditis: A study of four patients. *J.A.M.A.* 264:2916, 1990.
44. Grodzicki, R.L., and Steere, A.C. Comparison of immunoblotting and indirect enzyme-linked immunosorbent assay using different antigen preparations for diagnosing early Lyme disease. *J. Infect. Dis.* 157:790, 1988.
45. Craft, J.E., Fischer, D.K., Schimamato, G.T., and Steere, A.C. Antigens of *Borrelia burgdorferi* recognized during Lyme disease: Appearance of a new immunoglobulin M response and expansion of the immunoglobulin G response late in the illness. *J. Clin. Invest.* 78:934, 1986.
46. Hanrahan, J.P., Benach, J.L., Coleman, J.L., et al. Incidence and cumulative frequency of endemic Lyme disease in a community. *J. Infect. Dis.* 150:489, 1984.
47. Steere, A.C., Taylor, E., Wilson, M.L., et al. Longitudinal assessment of the clinical and epidemiological features of Lyme disease in a defined population. *J. Infect. Dis.* 154:295, 1986.
48. Stiernstedt, G.T., Granström, M., Hederstedt, B., and Sköldenberg, B. Diagnosis of spirochetal meningitis by enzyme-linked immunosorbent assay and indirect immunofluorescent assay in serum and cerebrospinal fluid. *J. Clin. Microbiol.* 21:819, 1985.
49. Dattwyler, R.J., Volkman, D.J., Luft, B.J., et al. Seronegative Lyme disease: Dissociation of specific T- and B-lymphocyte responses to *Borrelia burgdorferi*. *N. Engl. J. Med.* 319:1441, 1988.
50. Schutzer, S.E., Coyle, P.K., Belman, A.L., et al. Sequestration of antibody to *Borrelia burgdorferi* in immune complexes in seronegative Lyme disease. *Lancet* 1:312, 1990.
51. Rahn, D.W., and Malawista, S.E. Lyme disease: Recommendations for diagnosis and treatment. *Ann. Intern. Med.* 114:472, 1991.
52. Berger, B.W. Treatment of erythema chronicum migrans of Lyme disease. *Ann. N.Y. Acad. Sci.* 539:346, 1988.
53. Dattwyler, R.J., Volkman, D.J., Conaty, S.M., et al. Amoxicillin plus probenecid versus doxycycline for treatment of erythema migrans borreliosis. *Lancet* 1:1404, 1990.
54. Steere, A.C., Green, J., Hutchinson, G.J., et al. Treatment of Lyme disease. *Zentralbl. Bakteriol. Mikrobiol. Hyg. [A]* 236:352, 1986.
55. Weber, K., Preac-Mursic, V., Neubert, U., et al. Antibiotic therapy of early European Lyme borreliosis and acrodermatitis chronica atrophicans. *Ann. N.Y. Acad. Sci.* 539:324, 1988.

56. Steere, A.C., Pachner, A.R., and Malawista, S.E. Neurologic abnormalities of Lyme disease: Successful treatment with high-dose intravenous penicillin. *Ann. Intern. Med.* 99:767, 1983.
57. Dattwyler, R.J., Halperin, J.J., Volkman, D.J., and Luft, B.J. Treatment of late Lyme borreliosis—Randomized comparison of ceftriaxone and penicillin. *Lancet* 1:1191, 1988.

13

Thomas R. Swift

Fatigue in Neuromuscular Transmission Disorders

While many neurologic disorders are characterized by weakness, only neuromuscular transmission disorders are characterized by fatigue [1]. Fatigue in this context is narrowly defined as variability in muscle strength with worsening in relationship to exercise. This brief account of neuromuscular transmission disorders is included to serve as a basis for comparison with the more encompassing fatigue of the chronic fatigue syndrome (CFS).

PATHOGENESIS

The two major forms of neuromuscular blockade are both autoimmune. Myasthenia gravis is caused by formation of antireceptor antibodies [2]. Lambert-Eaton syndrome, which has a prevalence about one-fiftieth that of myasthenia, is caused by an antibody directed against voltage-gated calcium channels on the presynaptic side of the neuromuscular junction. The clinical features of myasthenia are discussed in the following section.

By contrast, several types of childhood, infantile, and congenital myasthenia exist that are not immunologic in origin. They may involve defects of receptor assembly or release, or abnormalities in acetylcholine-induced ion channel functions. All are very rare.

Botulinum intoxication also causes neuromuscular blockade at the level of the junction. The blockade is irreversible and causes loss of the blocked junctional apparatus. Recovery requires resynthesis of new neuromuscular junctions, which in humans can occur over a period of several months.

These illnesses are relevant to CFS in the sense that they may occasionally be considered as alternative diagnoses. Their pathogenesis differs in major ways, and other chapters in this book outline the evidence that fatigue as a symptom of CFS is usually attributable to an abnormality of the central nervous system. Some cases may be confusing, however. Patients with CFS may report muscle weakness, the examination may suggest an inconsistent muscular effort or weakness, and an examiner may not be certain of the basis for the complaint. CFS patients are more likely to report weakness than fatigue, and will usually state that their muscles weaken with use. By contrast, some patients with Lambert-Eaton syndrome have a paradoxical increase in strength after muscle contraction; this is noticed by some patients, detectable on testing in a few others, and often demonstrable by repetitive nerve stimulation in the electromyography laboratory. Fairly marked muscular atrophy, especially of larger proximal muscles, may occur in some patients with myasthenia. Tendon reflexes usually are absent in Lambert-Eaton syndrome. These findings will readily demonstrate that the peripheral nervous system is the site of the problem in the neuromuscular transmission disorders.

CLINICAL SYMPTOMS

For centuries, myasthenia gravis patients have been known to experience muscle weakness that varies dramatically, often over short periods of time: It is not infrequent that a patient admitted the night before with severely weak facial, shoulder, and neck muscles appears nearly normal on the following morning's rounds. Clinical findings easily demonstrate the fatigue. While speaking, words become progressively less distinct as though the tip of the tongue is hanging up between the teeth. While looking upward for a sustained period, the eyelid slowly moves down to cover the pupil. The arms, after being held outstretched for 20 seconds, begin to sag downward. A single deep knee bend is performed easily, while the fourth cannot be done at all. On sustained lateral gaze, progressive diplopia occurs. Chewing at first is vigorous but later must be assisted by the hand moving the mandible. During the day the facial appearance progressively assumes a myasthenic snarl. After a fit of coughing, dyspnea occurs. Progressive vital capacity measurements decline precipitously from normal or near normal levels. The first few stairs are climbed easily, the next slowly, the last laboriously. Patients report that they swallow their most important pills first because they know they may not get the others down.

To restore strength, patients learn the value of rest [3]. In the shower, periods of rest interrupt the shampoo. An afternoon nap is helpful, later essential, then a morning nap is introduced. Eating, drinking, and speaking are interrupted. Dressing, walking, stair climbing, hair combing, teeth brushing, and cooking can be done only for short periods. Increased body temperature may exacerbate the weakness.

The effect of medication may be dramatic [4]. Forty minutes after taking 60 mg of pyridostigmine bromide, strength improves. The facial appearance is pleasant, the head need not be propped up, ptosis disappears, double objects become single, a piece of sirloin can be swallowed, a key previously stuck in a lock can be turned, a jar lid is no longer too tight to open. Nasal regurgitation of liquids stops. The breathless nasal voice becomes clear and strong. A sag occurs 3½ hours later.

PATHOPHYSIOLOGY

Myasthenia gravis is a disease mediated by autoantibodies produced against nicotinic acetylcholine receptor protein [2]. Muscle end plates are destroyed by complement fixation, antigenic modulation, internalization of receptor, and finally simplification of postjunctional elements in which the numbers of viable acetylcholine receptors are drastically reduced [2]. Receptor blockade by antibody also occurs [2]. The muscle responds by upregulating receptor synthesis. The newly formed receptors are subsequently targeted for destruction; the balance between new production and destruction of receptor determines the patient's clinical state. Worsening of the patient's condition is undoubtedly antibody mediated, but all the factors inducing crisis are unknown. Such factors may include medication, receptor desensitization [5–7], presynaptic acetylcholine depletion [1], and other events.

Although virtually all evidence points to presynaptic events being normal in myasthenia gravis, the usual variations in the amount of released acetylcholine resulting from previous expenditures for exercise or nerve stimulation produce fluctuating weakness. Acetylcholine is synthesized in the nerve terminal, packaged, and released. It diffuses across the primary synaptic cleft where it attaches to receptor and produces end-plate potentials sufficiently large to reach threshold for muscle action potentials and cause the muscle to contract [1]. Much of the released acetylcholine is hydrolyzed by acetylcholinesterase, which renders it inert. Therefore, prevention of hydrolysis using anticholinesterase medications is a mainstay of treatment [4]. Overtreatment with anticholinesterase drugs results in continued stimulation of receptors, which may cause repetitive firing of the nerve and muscle and theoretically could produce acetylcholine-mediated receptor blockade with resultant increase in muscle weakness. However, it is questionable whether such "cholinergic crises" actually occur. The number of documented examples is small, and most patients who experience worsening do so because of progressive myasthenia, even if they are unresponsive to additional anticholinesterase agents.

Mechanisms of Fatigue

There are two mechanisms of fatigue in myasthenia gravis, and both remain incompletely understood. The first, and probably of lesser importance clinically, is the fatigue occurring during a period of exercise [1]. This is readily observed clinically as, for example, when the eyelid is unable to remain elevated during sustained upward gaze. The electrophysiologic correlate of this type of fatigue is the progressive reduction in muscle action potential amplitude during a train of stimuli.

A more subtle, yet probably more important type of fatigue in myasthenia gravis is what was originally termed "post-tetanic exhaustion" (better called *postactivation exhaustion*) [3]. This type of fatigue occurs following exercise after a latent period and probably accounts for the fatigue experienced by patients at the end of the day. The electrophysiologic correlate of this type of fatigue is the reduction in muscle action potential amplitude and increased decrement occurring maximally 2 to 4 minutes after exercise. Loss of the presynaptic transmitter stores expended during the exercise and loss of the facilitation that normally occurs immediately following exercise probably account for these changes. Facilitation is a complex phenomenon related to increased mobilization to release sites of vesicles containing acetylcholine [8] and the effect of calcium ions on facilitation release [9,10]. However, these transient phenomena serve to obscure the fact that transmitter stores have been depleted in the nerve terminal during exercise and because of this, acetylcholine output is decreased after the brief period of facilitation is over. The stores are eventually replenished through synthesis and packaging. These two phenomena, facilitation and exhaustion, may be observed clinically. In a patient with ptosis, a brief (30-second) period of sustained upgaze may cause improvement in the lid ptosis or even lid retraction for 15 to 30 seconds, whereas 2 minutes after the upgaze the ptosis is worse than before exercise even though no additional exercise has occurred.

TREATMENT

Symptomatic treatment of fatigue in myasthenia gravis involves rest, avoidance of repetitive muscle activity, avoidance of heat, and use of anticholinesterase, and stimulant drugs. In most patients, immunotherapy also is given to affect the underlying disease process [2].

Periods of rest not only provide a feeling of well-being, but allow time for acetylcholine stores to be replenished after activity. Fatiguing exercise causes expenditures of acetylcholine quanta, which are ultimately hydrolyzed by cholinesterase. Some of the choline liberated by hydrolysis is taken up into the nerve terminal and resynthesized into acetylcholine by the enzyme choline acetyltransferase. The acetylcholine is packaged into vesicles and eventually moved to release sites [1]. These processes take time. Because acetylcholine release at the nerve terminal is dependent on the number of quanta available for release multiplied by the probability of release, an increase in quanta at the release sites by itself increases the size of the end plate potential and reduces the likelihood of transmission failure [1]. Likewise, repetitive muscle activity reduces transmitter stores in affected muscles and should be avoided. Myasthenia patients report increased weakness with fever, in a hot bath or shower, or when exposed to high environmental temperatures. Heat probably worsens neuromuscular transmission by increasing the action of acetylcholinesterase, but it may also act to decrease the open time of the ion channel, increase the rate of receptor desensitization [6], or increase surrounding muscle membrane resistance, making it more difficult to translate a borderline end plate potential into a muscle action potential.

Anticholinesterase drugs, primarily pyridostigmine bromide (Mestinon), are the mainstay of treatment, reversibly inhibiting cholinesterase and allowing the normally released acetylcholine to attach to a greater percentage of the reduced number of receptors. Patients report improvement of strength about 40 minutes after a dose and often become weak and fatigued again about three hours later when nearly ready to take the next dose, but great variability occurs. When anticholinesterase drugs are abruptly discontinued, maximum weakness often does not occur until 36 to 48 hours later for reasons that are unclear. The drug also produces muscarinic effects of abdominal cramps and diarrhea, which are not an indication to reduce the dose. Instead, a muscarinic blocking drug, either oral atropine or tincture of belladonna, should be given to control muscarinic effects while the anticholinesterase treatment is continued. My practice is to give 8 to 10 drops of tincture of belladonna once daily in the morning fruit juice. The dosage can be titrated up if diarrhea continues or down if constipation supervenes.

A typical dose of pyridostigmine bromide is in the range of 60 to 180 mg three or four times per day. Overstimulation of nicotinic acetylcholine receptors can occur if too much pyridostigmine is given, manifested by diffuse fasciculations and cramps. Rarely does cholinergic block occur; treatment is withholding of the drug and reinstituting later at a lower dose. A long-acting form of pyridostigmine bromide is available.

Occasionally nonspecific stimulants are reported to be of benefit by patients. My practice is to use ephedrine 25 mg three times per day for symptomatic relief.

REFERENCES

1. Swift, T.R. Disorders of neuromuscular transmission other than myasthenia gravis. *Muscle Nerve* 4:334, 1981.
2. Drachman, D.B. Myasthenia gravis. *N. Engl. J. Med.* 298:136, 186, 1978.
3. Desmedt, J.E. Nature of the defect of neuromuscular transmission in myasthenic patients: "Post-tetanic exhaustion." *Nature* 179:156, 1957.
4. Walker, M.B. Treatment of myasthenia gravis with physostigmine. *Lancet* 1:1200, 1934.
5. Katz, B., Thesleff, S. A study of the "desensitization" produced by acetylcholine at the motor endplate. *J. Physiol.* 138:63, 1957.
6. Magayanik, L.G., Vyskocil, F. The effect of temperature on desensitization kinetics at the postsynaptic membrane of the frog muscle fiber. *J. Physiol.* 249:285, 1975.
7. Pagala, M.K.D., Namba, T., and Grob, D. Desensitization to acetylcholine at motor endplates in normal humans, patients with myasthenia gravis and experimental models of myasthenia gravis. *Ann. N.Y. Acad. Sci.* 377:567, 1981.
8. Wilson, D.F. Depression, facilitation, and mobilization of transmitter at the rat neuromuscular junction. *Am. J. Physiol.* 237:C31, 1979.
9. Katz, B., and Miledi, R. The role of calcium in neuromuscular facilitation. *J. Physiol.* 195:481, 1968.
10. Younkin, S.G. An analysis of the role of calcium in facilitation at the frog neuromuscular junction. *J. Physiol.* 237:1, 1974.

14

Nelson Gantz

Management of a Patient with Chronic Fatigue Syndrome

Chronic fatigue syndrome (CFS) is a disorder characterized by severe fatigue along with a group of specific symptoms and signs. Because the cause is unknown, specific therapy directed at the etiologic agent(s) is unavailable. However, much can be done to alleviate symptoms of the disorder in a group of individuals who are often frustrated and feel abandoned by traditional health care providers. This feeling of rejection often results in patients' seeking exotic, untested regimens from a group of practitioners for whom profit rather than science is the driving force. This chapter focuses on a rational approach to managing CFS so desperate patients can avoid untested alternative therapies, such as herbal remedies or colonic irrigation, which are potentially harmful.

TREATMENT STRATEGIES

Table 14-1 outlines treatment strategies that can be used to manage patients with CFS. While there are no specific treatments, establishing the diagnosis using the Centers for Disease Control case definition criteria is extremely beneficial to the patient [1]. Because no laboratory test exists to confirm the diagnosis, a careful and complete history is key. Once the diagnosis is made, it is important to provide emotional support for the patient and family as well as to educate the patient regarding what is known about this illness. Patients readily become misinformed

Table 14-1. Treatment strategies

Establish the diagnosis
Provide emotional support
Avoid exotic, unproved remedies
Provide symptomatic relief for:
  Depression
  Sleep disturbance
  Myalgias and arthralgias with nonsteroidal anti-inflammatory agents
  Allergies with nonsedating antihistamines
Continue to exclude other causes for patients' symptoms and signs
Avoid physical deconditioning using a graded exercise program and
  cognitive-behavior therapy
Refer patients to support groups
Provide regular follow-up every 4 to 6 weeks

as a result of a confusing array of anecdotes published in the lay press. It is vital to advise patients to avoid untested remedies. Some of these agents and approaches are listed in Table 14-2. These drugs can be harmful and costly, and most have not been subject to controlled scientific trials.

A selected number of agents have been studied in a controlled manner, and they are listed in Table 14-3 and described here.

Acyclovir

Since the majority of patients report a viral-like illness at the onset, it is not surprising that acyclovir was used in the first controlled trial to treat patients with CFS [2]. Acyclovir is active against herpesviruses such as Epstein-Barr virus (EBV), the virus initially implicated as the causative agent in this disorder [3,4]. In a well-designed placebo-controlled study involving 27 subjects taking high-dose intravenous acyclovir, Straus et al. found that about 40% of patients in both the placebo- and drug-treated groups responded [2]. Acyclovir was also associated with reversible renal failure in 12% of the acyclovir-treated patients [2]. Immunologic tests and EBV serologic assays were unaffected by the acyclovir.

Liver Extract

In a controlled trial involving 15 patients with CFS, intramuscular injection of a mixture of bovine liver extract, folic acid, and cyanocobalamin produced a similar response rate compared with placebo for patients with the disorder [5]. Interestingly, in an earlier trial by the same authors using an open label format, 100% of the patients showed a dramatic response to this material. That result emphasizes the importance of

Table 14-2. Selected agents and approaches that have been used to treat CFS

ACE inhibitors	Antidepressants
Captopril	Tricyclic antidepressants
Enalapril	Amitriptyline
Antibacterials	Desipramine
Ceftriaxone	Doxepin
Ciprofloxacin	Fluoxetine
Doxycycline	Nortriptyline
Fusidic acid	MAOIs
Antifungals	Phenelzine
Ketoconazole	Others
Nystatin	Lithium
Antihistamines	Buspirone
H_2-receptor blockers	Stimulants
Anti-inflammatory drugs	Amphetamines
Hydroxychloroquine	Vitamins/minerals
NSAIDs	Cyanocobalamin
Antivirals	Ascorbic acid
Acyclovir	Zinc
Calcium-channel blockers	Magnesium sulfate
Nifedipine	Other agents
Immune modifiers	Germanium
Ampligen	Kutapressin
Corticosteroids	Primrose oil
Cyclophosphamide	Vasopressin
Immune globulin	Herbs
Interferon-α	Essential fatty acids
Interleukin-2	Other approaches
Isoprinosine (inosine pranobex)	Anti-candida diets
Pentoxifylline	Ingestion of yogurt and cultures of
Thymic extract	lactobacilli
Transfer factor	Acupuncture
Opium antagonist	Royal jelly
Naltrexone	Colonic irrigation
Psychoactive agents	Cognitive-behavior therapy
Anxiolytics	Hypnosis
Benzodiazepines	Graded exercise
Carbamazepine	Transcendental meditation
Clonazepam	Hydrotherapy
Alprazolam	Removal of dental fillings

ACE = angiotensin-converting enzyme; NSAIDs = nonsteroidal anti-inflammatory drugs; MAOIs = monoamine oxidase inhibitors.
Source: Modified from Gantz and Holmes [20] and McBride and McCluskey [14].

performing double-blind randomized controlled trials before advocating any of these so-called miracle cures.

Immune Globulin

Based on the theory that patients with CFS have an immunoregulatory

Table 14-3. Selected agents that have been
studied in a controlled manner to treat CFS

Acyclovir
Liver extract, folic acid, vitamin B_{12}
Immune globulin (intravenous)
Magnesium sulfate
Essential fatty acids
Amitriptyline (low dose)[a]
Amitriptyline and naproxen[a]
Cyclobenzaprine[a]
Ibuprofen and alprazolam[a]

---

[a]For patients with fibromyalgia.

deficit, immune globulin has been administered to patients with the disorder. One uncontrolled study involving 19 patients reported a beneficial effect from intramuscular immune globulin [6]. Numerous anecdotes also attest to favorable responses obtained in patients with CFS given intravenous immunoglobulin. Building on this background of information, two controlled studies using high-dose intravenous immunoglobulin were conducted that reached conflicting conclusions about the therapeutic benefit.

One well-designed controlled study conducted in the United States, involving 28 adults given 1 gm/kg of intravenous immunoglobulin or placebo, noted no difference in response rates in the two groups [7]. Patients received monthly infusions for 6 months, and about 20% in each group reported symptomatic improvement. In the other well-designed controlled trial, in Australia, the investigators treated 49 adults with either 2 gm/kg of immunoglobulin or placebo for 3 months. In this study, 43% of recipients given immunoglobulin reported feeling better compared with 12% of those given placebo infusions [8]. The symptomatic improvement was noted only at 3 months after the final infusion, and in those who responded, symptoms and disability returned 6 months after the end of therapy. Some of the patients who responded and then relapsed were again treated with intravenous immunoglobulin, resulting in remission of symptoms and functional improvement. Adverse effects of immunoglobulin therapy included phlebitis (55%) and constitutional symptoms (82%) such as headaches, fatigue, and diminished concentration that persisted up to 10 days after the infusion [8].

Why there was a difference in outcome in these two well-designed studies is unclear. Possible factors include: (1) smaller sample size in the U.S. study, (2) lower dose of immunoglobulin in the U.S. study, (3) different study populations, and (4) different methods of assessing outcome in the two studies [9]. At present, intravenous immune globulin cannot be recommended because of its cost, and further studies are warranted to resolve this issue.

Magnesium Sulfate

Investigators in England noted that patients with CFS had diminished red blood cell magnesium levels [10]. In a double-blind randomized trial of intramuscular magnesium sulfate (1 gm in 2 ml) weekly for 6 weeks, 80% of patients given magnesium injections had improved energy levels and less pain compared with 18% of the subjects given placebo. After treatment, red blood cell magnesium levels returned to normal in all patients given magnesium. Another investigator in the United States was unable to confirm the diminished red blood cell magnesium levels in patients with CFS [11]. The possible benefits of intramuscular magnesium sulfate injections must be confirmed since the only follow-up was at 6 weeks.

Essential Fatty Acids

Essential fatty acids have antiviral activity and decrease cytokine production [12]. Behan et al. conducted a prospective randomized, double-blind trial of a mixture of essential fatty acids or placebo for a 3-month period [13]. Patients received 1 gm per day of a mixture of oil of evening primrose and fish oil. At 3 months, 85% of treated patients improved compared with 17% of the placebo group. In another well-controlled trial, there was no difference in the response rate between those given active treatment versus placebo [14]. Further data are needed to clarify this issue, and long-term results of essential fatty acid therapy are unknown.

Amitriptyline and Other Agents

Sleep disturbance and depression are prominent symptoms in patients with CFS. Tricyclic antidepressants such as amitriptyline are often beneficial. In a randomized 6-week trial of 25 mg of amitriptyline or placebo at bedtime, patients with fibromyalgia noted improved sleep, less pain, and diminished fatigue [15]. Amitriptyline in doses as low as 10 mg may be effective in patients with CFS. In the same study, the combination of amitriptyline (25 mg) plus naproxen (500 mg twice daily) was more effective than placebo. Naproxen alone, however, was no better than placebo.

The long-term effectiveness of various tricyclic antidepressants as well as the optimal nonsteroidal anti-inflammatory drug (NSAID) are unknown. In another trial, cyclobenzaprine in doses from 20 to 40 mg at bedtime for 12 weeks was effective in decreasing pain, improving sleep, and diminishing fatigue in patients with fibromyalgia [16,17]. Because of the similarity of fibromyalgia and CFS, patients with CFS should benefit from a trial of low-dose amitriptyline plus an NSAID. Response usually occurs in 3 to 4 weeks.

TREATMENT OF DEPRESSION

Depression occurs frequently in patients with CFS, and it is reasonable to try an antidepressant in patients with this disorder [18,19]. Use of an antidepressant does not imply that the patient has a psychiatric illness, nor does a response to a drug indicate that depression and not CFS is the diagnosis. Patients with CFS and depression should be treated with full-dose antidepressant therapy, using an agent that is effective and that the patient can tolerate [20]. The choice of agents depends on the patient's symptoms and the drug's adverse effects. Drugs should be given for a 4- to 6-week period before considering them a therapeutic failure.

Anecdotally, patients who complain of difficulty falling asleep or staying asleep at night may gain greater benefits from the more sedating agents such as amitriptyline or doxepin. Sedating drugs are best taken 2 hours before bedtime. The adverse side effects of tricyclic agents, such as their anticholinergic effects, may resolve with continuation of therapy. Another highly sedating drug is trazodone, which has minimal anticholinergic effects. Its main problems are postural hypotension and nausea. Imipramine is a tricyclic agent with mild sedative effects, and tricyclics with even less sedation include desipramine, nortriptyline, and protriptyline. Cardiac conduction system disease is the major contraindication to the use of tricyclics.

Another class of antidepressants is the monoamine oxidase inhibitors (MAOIs) such as phenelzine. While these agents are effective as antidepressants, the serious potential adverse effects related to various interactions with foods containing tyramine, phenylalanine, dopamine, and similar chemicals make their use difficult to justify. There are no controlled studies using MAOI drugs, but only favorable anecdotal experience.

Another antidepressant, bupropion, may be beneficial in CFS for selected patients, but agitation and seizures may occur. Bupropion should be taken in the morning.

Fluoxetine is an extremely effective drug for depression in patients with CFS. The drug is stimulating and must be taken in the morning, or at noon if the patient cannot tolerate a single dose in the morning. Dosage of fluoxetine is from 20 to 60 mg once a day. If a patient cannot tolerate the 20 mg capsule, half of the dose can be tried. Fluoxetine is water soluble, making the lower dose easy to administer. Again, no controlled studies are available using fluoxetine for patients with CFS.

TREATMENT OF ANXIETY AND PANIC DISORDERS

Anxiety and panic attacks may occur in patients with CFS. Drugs such as clonazepam (Klonopin), alprazolam (Xanax), or buspirone (BuSpar) may be useful for anxiety. Alprazolam is particularly helpful in blocking panic attacks. The major disadvantage of alprazolam is that it is potentially habit forming and requires a dosage schedule of three to four times a day because of its short half-life. While some physicians consider the psychiatric symptoms in patients with CFS to be the cause of the disorder, others view them as a reaction to the illness. It is clearly beneficial to treat patients' symptoms and avoid an attitude of mind/body dualism [21].

TREATMENT OF ALLERGIES

Allergies are common in patients with CFS. In one report, atopy was noted in more than 50% of patients with the disorder [22]. Many patients report allergies to inhalants, food, or drugs. There is no evidence that food-elimination diets are helpful in patients with CFS. Nonsedating antihistamines such as terfenadine (Seldane) or astemizole (Hismanal) can be tried, but no controlled studies are available. Nystatin therapy was no better than placebo for patients with the so-called yeast connection, or candida hypersensitivity syndrome [23].

TREATMENT OF MYALGIAS AND ARTHRALGIAS

Myalgias, particularly involving the neck and shoulder muscles though others may be involved as well, occur frequently, as do arthralgias. Arthritis is not a feature of CFS and, if present, should suggest another diagnosis. As noted, NSAIDs may be used for the pain. In one controlled study, the combination of ibuprofen and alprazolam was effective in treating patients with fibromyalgia [24]. The dosage for ibuprofen was 2.4 gm daily and that for alprazolam, 0.5 to 3.0 mg daily. Patients noted a significant decrease in pain compared with the placebo [24].

The headaches and fever may also respond to NSAIDs. Corticosteroids should be avoided. In one controlled trial, prednisolone 10 to 60 mg per day was tried and found ineffective. Some patients' illnesses actually became worse after a 2-month course of steroid therapy [25].

TREATMENT OF PHYSICAL DECONDITIONING

Many patients with CFS avoid activity because characteristically it often results in recurrence of symptoms with exacerbation of fever, fatigue, and myalgias. This behavior eventually leads to a vicious cycle of deconditioning, resulting in even less activity. Some success has been achieved using a combination of graded exercise therapy and cognitive-behavior therapy. It must be emphasized that the exercise should be *gradual* and vigorous activity should be avoided initially.

Cognitive-behavior or learning therapy refers to the use of techniques to change behavior by altering a patient's attitudes, perceptions, and belief systems. This approach focuses on modifying an individual's attitudes regarding the symptoms, in contrast to direct treatment of specific symptoms [26]. Cognitive-behavior therapy was found to be effective in reducing symptoms and increasing activity in patients with fibromyalgia [27]. In one uncontrolled trial of cognitive-behavior therapy in CFS, 69% of the patients had improved functioning and noted a decrease in symptoms at a 3-month follow-up [26]. Depressed patients responded poorly. Unfortunately, there was no control group and 36% of the patients did not participate in the trial.

ADVICE FOR THE PATIENT

In the absence of a specific therapeutic agent, patients with CFS should be instructed to modify their life-style as much as possible. They should eat a balanced diet and get sufficient rest. There is no evidence that prolonged rest is curative. As noted, *gradual* exercise should be encouraged. Patients must learn to pace themselves and set realistic new personal goals. Physical and emotional stress should be avoided as much as possible because these factors may exacerbate the illness.

Once the diagnosis of CFS is made, it is important for the physician to continue to exclude other causes for the patient's symptoms and signs. Patients need reassurance and compassion, and their complaints must be taken seriously despite normal results on routine laboratory studies. Patients should be instructed that the disorder is not progressive but tends to wax and wane in severity. Counseling and support groups may help patients and families cope with the symptoms as well as the often devastating economic consequences of loss of employment. Instruction in techniques to reduce stress may be invaluable.

The prognosis for complete recovery is unknown, and studies are needed to document the natural history of this illness. Anecdotally, approximately 20% of patients spontaneously get better. Patients who report their illness as having a discrete onset and deny prior psychiatric illness tend to do better than those reporting a gradual onset who have a positive past psychiatric history. Physicians should provide their patients regular follow-up visits every 4 to 6 months.

CONCLUSION

Further controlled studies are needed to evaluate various treatments to alleviate the symptoms of CFS. A promising compound is ampligen, or poly (I) : poly (C 12 U). This drug is a mismatched double-stranded RNA that is hypothesized to enhance the immune system. The results of a preliminary unpublished study with ampligen showed significant relief of symptoms compared with placebo after 24 weeks of therapy. Data on the adverse effects and long-term benefits of ampligen therapy in a well-controlled study are needed.

REFERENCES

1. Holmes, G.P., Kaplan, J.E., Gantz, N.M., et al. Chronic fatigue syndrome: A working case definition. *Ann. Intern. Med.* 108:387, 1988.
2. Straus, S.E., Dale, J.K., Tobi, M., et al. Acyclovir treatment of the chronic fatigue syndrome. *N. Engl. J. Med.* 319:1692, 1988.
3. Jones, J.F., Ray, C.F., Minnich, L.L., et al. Evidence for active Epstein-Barr virus infection in patients with persistent, unexplained illnesses: elevated anti-early antigen antibodies. *Ann. Intern. Med.* 102:7, 1985.
4. Straus, S.E., Tosato, G., Armstrong, G., et al. Persisting illness and fatigue in adults with evidence of Epstein-Barr virus infection. *Ann. Intern. Med.* 102:7, 1985.
5. Kaslow, J.E., Rucker, L., and Onishi, R. Liver extract–folic acid–cyanocobalamin vs placebo for chronic fatigue syndrome. *Arch. Intern. Med.* 149:2501, 1989.
6. DuBois, R.E. Gamma globulin therapy for chronic mononucleosis syndrome. *AIDS Res.* 2:S191, 1986.
7. Peterson, P.K., Shepard, J., Macres, M., et al. A controlled trial of intravenous immunoglobulin G in chronic fatigue syndrome. *Am. J. Med.* 89:554, 1990.
8. Lloyd, A., Hickie, I., Wakefield, D., et al. A double-blind, placebo-controlled trial of intravenous immunoglobulin therapy in patients with chronic fatigue syndrome. *Am. J. Med.* 89:561, 1990.
9. Straus, S.E. Intravenous immunoglobulin treatment for the chronic fatigue syndrome. *Am. J. Med.* 89:551, 1990.
10. Cox, I.M., Campbell, M.J., Dowson, D. Red blood cell magnesium and chronic fatigue syndrome. *Lancet* 337:757, 1991.
11. Gantz, N.M. Magnesium and chronic fatigue. *Lancet* 338:66, 1991.
12. Endres, S., Ghorbani, R., Kelley, V.E., et al. The effect of dietary supplementation with n-3 polyunsaturated fatty acids on the synthesis of interleukin-1 and tumor necrosis factor by mononuclear cells. *N. Engl. J. Med.* 302:265, 1989.
13. Behan, P.O., Behan, W.M.H., and Horrobin, D. Effect of high doses of essential fatty acids on the postviral fatigue syndrome. *Acta Neurol. Scand.* 82:209, 1990.
14. McBride, S.J., and McCluskey, D.R. Treatment of chronic fatigue syndrome. *Br. Med. Bull.* 47:895, 1991.
15. Goldenberg, D.L., Felson, D.T., and Dinerman, H. A randomized, controlled trail of amitriptyline and naproxen in the treatment of patients with fibromyalgia. *Arthritis Rheum.* 29:1371, 1986.
16. Bennett, R.M., Gatter, R.A., Campbell, S.M., et al. A comparison of cyclobenzaprine and placebo in the management of fibrositis. *Arthritis Rheum.* 31:1535, 1988.
17. Goldenberg, M.D. Fibromyalgia, chronic fatigue syndrome, and myofascial pain syndrome. *Curr. Opin. Rheum.* 3:247, 1991.

18. Manu, P., Lane, T.J., and Matthews, D.A. The frequency of the chronic fatigue syndrome in patients with symptoms of persistent fatigue. *Ann. Intern. Med.* 109:554, 1988.
19. Manu, P., Matthews, D., and Lane, T. The mental health of patients with a chief complaint of chronic fatigue. *Arch. Intern. Med.* 148:2213, 1988.
20. Gantz, N.M., and Holmes, G.P. Treatment of patients with chronic fatigue syndrome. *Drugs* 38:855, 1989.
21. Komaroff, A.L. The chronic fatigue syndrome. *Ann. Intern. Med.* 110:407, 1989.
22. Straus, S.E., Dale, J.K., Wright, R., and Metcalfe, D.D. The chronic fatigue syndrome. *J. Allergy Clin. Immunol.* 81:791, 1988.
23. Dismukes, W.E., Wade, J.S., Lee, J.Y., et al. A randomized double-blind trial of nystatin therapy for the candidiasis hypersensitivity syndrome. *N. Engl. J. Med.* 323:1718, 1990.
24. Russell, I.J., Fletcher, E.M., Michalek, J.E., et al. Treatment of primary fibrositis/fibromyalgia syndrome with ibuprofen and alprozolam. *Arthritis Rheum.* 34:552, 1991.
25. Behan, P.O., and Behan, W.M.H. Postviral fatigue syndrome. *CRC Crit. Rev. Neurobiol.* 4:157, 1988.
26. Butler, S., Chalder, T., Ron, M., and Wessely, S. Cognitive behavior therapy in the chronic fatigue syndrome. *J. Neurol. Neurosurg. Psychiatry* 54:153, 1991.
27. McCain, G., Bell, D.A., Mai, F.M., and Halliday, P.D. A controlled study of the effects of a supervised cardiovascular fitness training programme on the manifestations of primary fibromyalgia. *Arthritis Rheum.* 31:1135, 1988.

15

David M. Dawson
Thomas D. Sabin

Summary and Perspective

Fatigue is a symptom of many physiologic states. It can be a response to intense physical effort, in which case it is a phenomenon of normal life. It can have a peripheral cause, as in myasthenia gravis or primary myopathy. It can be a symptom resulting from central nervous system disease, and is especially characteristic of multiple sclerosis. Patients with chronic illness outside the nervous system complain of feeling tired; this complaint seems especially common with autoimmune disease, chronic granulomas, and cancer. With depression, along with many other psychiatric symptoms, fatigue is reported.

No one can say at this point if these kinds of fatigue share a common pathogenesis. One can imagine that a patient with Parkinson's disease who complains of fatigue is reporting some mismatch between effort and accomplishment: He is defeated by rigidity or akinesia. A patient with fever and weight loss due to lymphoma reports fatigue; surely she must be telling us something about circulating cytokines, about products of cell necrosis, or about metabolic derangements due to tumor growth. Many of these issues are touched on in the preceding chapters. For a skeptical view of fatigue, chronic fatigue syndrome (CFS), and psycho-somatic illness of other descriptions, Shorter's review may be consulted [1]. Here we would like to offer some provisional recommendations for a schedule of evaluation in suspected cases of CFS and to record our own ideas about possible causes of the syndrome.

EVALUATION OF
CHRONIC FATIGUE

History

1. Delineation of the primary complaint. Is the patient referring to muscular fatigue, that is, weakness? Is it slowness in initiation of movement? Does physical or mental effort bring it on? What about time of day, relationship to anxiety, effort, or other simultaneous somatic complaints? Some idea of the intensity of the fatigue can be gathered by estimating reduction in activities: Does the patient sleep or rest during the day? Come home early? Rest over the weekend rather than play golf? Careful documentation of daily activities will help diagnostically and in follow-up.

2. Associated psychiatric complaints. As pointed out by Wessely [2], fatigue is a common complaint in primary care medical practice, often associated with depression, anxiety, and lack of exercise. A survey reports that 14% of men and 20% of women report themselves to be significantly fatigued [3]. In the milder forms of depression seen in medical practice, depression and fatigue along with somatic symptoms such as headache, dizziness, palpitations, and dyspnea will often precede the typical psychiatric symptoms of major depression [2]. Only a few patients with persistent fatigue fulfill the criteria for CFS [4].

The evaluation of a fatigued patient must include thoughtful inquiry into a possible role of depression. Particular attention to prior episodes of depression may furnish an important (but not fully reliable) way to distinguish CFS from primary depression (see Chapter 3).

3. As with fatigue, an effort should be made to estimate the degree of cognitive disturbance present. Has the patient begun to use more lists? Forgotten appointments? Become lost while driving? Given up reading? Have others noted changes?

4. Patients whose illness adheres to research guidelines of the U.S. Centers for Disease Control [5] may have fever or feverishness, adenopathy, pharyngitis, myalgia, or arthralgia. They should not have true muscle weakness or signs of arthritis. Many (particularly in the epidemics) report paresthesias, which often are migratory. In some recent patients, transitory ataxia, gait disturbance, and asymptomatic reflex changes have been found [6]. Nevertheless, a history suggesting focal and fixed neurologic deficit is uncommon in CFS. The history should search for symptoms pointing away from the syndrome, such as abdominal pain, urinary incontinence, unilateral visual loss, weight loss, and similar complaints.

5. Medication history. We reproduce a list of drugs known to cause fatigue, courtesy of the staff of *Physicians' Desk Reference* (Table 15-1). No further comment is needed.

Table 15 1. Drugs known to cause fatigue (incidence)

A.P.L.
▲Accutane Capsules (Approximately 1 in 20)
Actifed with Codeine Cough Syrup
Actigall Capsules
Children's Advil Suspension
AeroBid Inhaler System (1–3%)
Ambenyl Cough Syrup
Amen
Amicar Intravenous, Syrup & Tablets
Ancobon Capsules
Antabuse (Small number of patients)
Asendin Tablets (Greater than 1%)
Atromid-S (Less often)
Atrovent Inhalation Aerosol (Less than 1%)
Azdone Tablets
Azo Gantrisin Tablets
Bactrim DS Tablets
Bactrim I.V. Infusion
Bactrim
Benadryl Capsules
Benadryl Kapseals
Benadryl Injection
▲Blocadren Tablets (3.4% to 5%)
Brevibloc Injection (1%)
Bumex (0.1%)
Buprenex Injectable (Less than 1%)
▲BuSpar (4%)
Calan SR Caplets (1.7%)
Calan Tablets (1.7%)
Capoten (0.5 to 2%)
Capozide (0.5 to 2%)
▲Cartrol Tablets (0.5–7.1%)
▲Catapres Tablets (About 4 in 100 patients)
▲Catapres-TTS (4% to 6%)
▲Centrax Capsules (11.6%)
Cesamet Pulvules
Choloxin
Cholybar
Cibalith-S Syrup
Clinoril Tablets (Less than 1 in 100)
Colestid Granules (1–3 patients in 1,000)
Combipres Tablets
Compazine
▲Cordarone Tablets (4 to 9%)
Corgard (2 in 100 patients)
Cortifoam
Corzide (2%)

Cosmegen Injection
Cycrin Tablets
Cytotec (Infrequent)
Danocrine
▲Dantrium Capsules (Among most frequent)
Deconamine
Demulen
Depo-Provera Sterile Aqueous Suspension (Occasional)
Desyrel and Desyrel Dividose (Greater than 1%)
Dibenzyline Capsules
▲Disopyramide Phosphate CR Capsules (3–9%)
Diulo
Dolobid Tablets (Greater than 1 in 100)
Doral Tablets (1.9%)
Dyazide Capsules
Dyrenium Capsules (Rare)
Edecrin
Elavil
Eldepryl
Elspar
Emete-con Intramuscular/ Intravenous
Empirin with Codeine Phosphate Nos. 2, 3 & 4 (Occasional)
Endep Tablets
Enovid
▲Epogen for Injection (9.0%)
Esimil Tablets
Eskalith
Etrafon
Fansidar Tablets
Feldene Capsules (Occasional)
Flexeril Tablets (1% to 3%)
Fulvicin P/G Tablets
Fulvicin P/G 165 & 330 Tablets
Fulvicin-U/F Tablets
Gantanol
Gantrisin
Grifulvin V (griseofulvin microsize) Tablets/Suspension (Occasional)
Grisactin (Occasional)
Grisactin Ultra (Occasional)
Gris-PEG Tablets, 125 mg & 250 mg (Occasional)
Halcion Tablets (Less frequent)
Heptavax-B (1.9%)
▲Hismanal Tablets (4.2%)
Humulin 70/30

Table 15-1. (continued)

Humulin BR, 100 Units
Humulin L, 100 Units
Humulin U Ultralente
Hydromox R Tablets
▲Hytrin Tablets (11.3%)
INH Tablets
IFEX (Less than 1%)
Immune Globulin, Intravenous
  (Human), Gammagard
  (Occasional)
Imodium Capsules
Inderal Injectable
Inderal LA Long Acting Capsules
Inderal Tablets
Inderide LA Long Acting Capsules
Inderide Tablets
Indocin (Greater than 1%)
▲Intron A (18% to 84%)
Inversine Tablets
Iopidine
Ismelin Tablets
Isoptin Injectable (Few)
Isoptin Oral Tablets (1.7%)
Isoptin SR Sustained Release
  Tablets (1.7%)
K-Lyte
K-Phos M.F. Tablets
K-Phos Neutral Tablets
K-Phos Original Formula 'Sodium
  Free' Tablets (Less frequent)
K-Phos No. 2 Tablets
Keflet Tablets
Keftab Tablets
Kenalog-10 Injection
Kenalog-40 Injection
Lamprene Capsules (Less than 1%)
Larodopa (Relatively frequent)
▲Levatol (4.4%)
Limbitrol
Lioresal Tablets (2–4%)
Lithium Carbonate Capsules &
  Tablets
Lithobid Tablets
▲Lopid Capsules and Tablets (3.8%)
▲Lopressor Ampuls (10%)
▲Lopressor HCT Tablets (10 in 100
  patients)
▲Lopressor (10%)
Lortab ASA Tablets (Occasional)
▲Lozol Tablets (Greater than or equal
  to 5%)
▲Ludiomil Tablets (4%)
Lupron Injection (Less than 5%)

▲Marplan Tablets (Among most
  frequent)
Matulane Capsules
Maxair Inhaler (Less than 1%)
Maxzide
Meclomen (Rare)
Mesantoin Tablets
▲Mesnex Injection (33%)
Methotrexate Tablets, Parenteral
  and LPF Parenteral (Frequent)
Metrodin (urofollitropin for
  injection) (Less than 1 in 50)
▲Mexitil Capsules (1.9% to 3.8%)
Midamor Tablets (Between 1% and
  3%)
Mintezol
Moduretic Tablets (Greater than 1%,
  less than 3%)
Motofen Tablets (1 in 200 to 1 in
  600)
Motrin Tablets
Mutamycin
▲Mykrox ½ mg Tablets (4.4%)
Myleran Tablets
Mysoline (Occasional)
Nalfon (Less than 3%)
Nardil (Common)
Navane Capsules and Concentrate
Navane Intramuscular
▲NebuPent for Inhalation Solution
  (53–72%)
Neptazane Tablets
▲Nolvadex Tablets (3.8% to 10%)
Norethin
Norlutate
Norlutin
Normodyne Injection
▲Normodyne Tablets (5%)
▲Normozide Tablets (1% to 5%)
Noroxin Tablets (0.3% to 1%)
▲Norpace (3 to 9%)
Norpramin Tablets
▲Octamide PFS (10% of patients)
Optimine Tablets
Ornade Spansule Capsules
PBZ Tablets & Elixir
PBZ-SR Tablets
Pamelor
Paradione Capsules & Oral Solution
▲Parlodel (1–7%)
Peganone Tablets
Pentaspan Injection
Pepcid (Infrequent)

Table 15-1. (continued)

Peptavion
Periactin
Phenergan Injection
Phenurone Tablets (Less than 1%)
Pipracil
Polaramine
Pondimin Tablets
Pregnyl
▲Prinivil Tablets (3.3%)
▲Prinzide Tablets (3.7%)
Profasi (human chorionic
  gonadotropin, USP)
Proventil Syrup (Children 2–6: 1%)
Provera Tablets
▲Prozac Pulvules (Most common)
Quadrinal Tablets
Questran Light
Questran Powder
Recombivax HB (Equal to or greater
  than 1%)
▲Reglan (10%)
Renese-R Tablets
Rheumatrex Methotrexate Dose
  Pack (Frequent)
RhoGAM Rh$_O$(D) Immune Globulin
  (Human)
Rifadin
Rifamate Capsules
Rimactane Capsules
▲Roferon-A Injection (89% to 95%)
Rogaine Topical Solution (0.28%)
▲Rowasa (3.44%)
Ru-Tuss II Capsules
Sandostatin Injection (1.4%)
Sansert Tablets
▲Sectral Capsules (11%)
▲Seldane Tablets (4.5%)
Septra
Septra I.V. Infusion
Septra I.V. Infusion ADD-Vantage
  Vials
Septra
Serophene (clomiphene citrate
  tablets, USP) (0.8%)
Sinemet Tablets
Sinequan (Occasional)
Stelazine
Stilphostrol Tablets and Ampuls
Surmontil Capsules
Symmetrel Capsules & Syrup (0.1–
  1%)
Tacaryl
▲Tambocor Tablets (7.7%)

Tavist Syrup
Tavist Tablets
Tavist-D Tablets
▲Tegison Capsules (50–75%)
Tegretol Chewable Tablets
Tegretol Suspension
Tegretol Tablets
Temaril Tablets, Syrup and
  Spansule Sustained Release
  Capsules
▲Tenex Tablets (3% to 4%)
▲Tenoretic Tablets (26%)
▲Tenormin Tablets (6%)
Thalitone Tablets
Timolide Tablets (1.9%)
Timoptic in Ocudose
Timoptic Sterile Ophthalmic
  Solution
Tofranil Ampuls
Tofranil Tablets
Tofranil-PM Capsules
Tolinase Tablets (Infrequent)
Tonocard Tablets (0.8–1.6%)
Trandate HCT Tablets (1% in 208
  patients)
Trandate Injection
▲Trandate Tablets (11%)
Tranxene
Trexan Tablets (Less than 1%)
Triaminic Expectorant DH
Triaminic Oral Infant Drops
Triaminic TR Tablets (Timed
  Release)
Triamterene & Hydrochlorothiazide
  Capsules
Triavil Tablets
Tridione
Trinalin Repetabs Tablets
Unasyn (Less than 1%)
Uroqid-Acid (Less frequent)
▲Valium Injectable (Among most
  common)
▲Valium Tablets (Among most
  common)
▲Valrelease Capsules (Among most
  common)
▲Vaseretic Tablets (3.9%)
Vasotec I.V. (0.5 to 1%)
Vasotec Tablets (1.8% to 3.0%)
Ventolin Syrup (1% of children)
▲Visken Tablets (8%)
Vivactil Tablets
Voltaren Tablets

Table 15-1. (continued)

▲Wellbutrin Tablets (5.0%)	Muscular
Xanax Tablets (Greater than 1%)	Demi-Regroton Tablets
Zarontin Capsules	Prinzide Tablets
Zarontin Syrup	Regroton Tablets
▲Zestoretic (3.7%)	Triamterene & Hydrochlorothiazide Capsules
▲Zestril Tablets (3.3%)	Zestoretic
Zovirax Capsules (0.3%)	

▲ = 3% incidence

Source: Copyright © *PDR Drug Interactions and Side Effects Index,* 1992 edition. Published by Medical Economics Data, Montvale, NJ 07654. (Used with permission.)

Laboratory Evaluation

Standard recommendations for laboratory testing would include the following [5]:

1. Complete blood count, electrolytes, calcium and phosphorus, total protein, serum protein electrophoresis, liver chemistry tests
2. Creatine kinase level (to exclude myopathy)
3. Sedimentation rate (to screen for vasculitis and cancer)
4. Antinuclear antibody, rheumatoid factor (point toward collagen vascular disease)
5. Thyroid-stimulating hormone (with or without tri-iodothyronine)
6. Human immunodeficiency virus serology (fatigue can be an early symptom of AIDS)
7. Epstein-Barr viral capsid antigen serology
8. Cytomegalovirus serology
9. Toxoplasma serology
10. VDRL
11. Lyme serology
12. Magnetic resonance imaging of the head (to exclude multiple sclerosis, a common confounding diagnosis; also to evaluate for the presence of pituitary disease and to check for scattered lesions that may be seen in some CFS patients)

Special studies that might be done in selected instances or in patients who are part of a study group include:

1. CD4 : CD8 T-cell ratio [7,8]
2. Activation antigens (e.g., CD38, HLA-DR) [7,8]
3. Natural killer (NK) cells [7]
4. Herpesvirus-6 [6] and HTLV [9] serology
5. Electroencephalogram with sleep study (see Chapter 10)
6. Neuropsychologic testing

7. Structured psychiatric interview (e.g., Diagnostic Interview Schedule of the National Institute of Mental Health) [10]
8. Nerve conduction/electromyographic testing, possibly including single-fiber electromyography (see Chapter 13)
9. Lumbar puncture
10. Muscle biopsy [11]

In each of these instances, there is documentation of an abnormality in some groups of research patients or significant differential diagnosis issues are known to occur. Because these examinations may not lead to a therapy, it is difficult to recommend them on a wide scale. The risk/benefit ratio in employing further testing needs to be carefully watched. Patients may become desperate as their devastating symptoms continue, and will turn to their physician hoping for definition or validation. Many will bring with them publications from lay or support organizations, several of which are excellent and contain up-to-date information (including publications from the Chronic Fatigue and Immune Dysfunction Syndrome Association in the United States and the British Myalgic Encephalomyelitis Association). Continuation of exhausting, painful, or expensive testing beyond a reasonable level is not warranted [12].

SPECULATIONS ON PATHOGENESIS

Neurologists by their training seek to establish a diagnosis that explains both the nature of an illness and its localization in one or more parts of the nervous system. CFS puzzles us on both counts. Only the most rudimentary information is available about what the illness is or where it is located. Possible explanations also need to account for these features, which seem common:

1. Epidemic nature of the illness in some instances.
2. A potential duration of many years. Some patients in the Akureyri epidemic in Iceland were still symptomatic, although no worse, many decades later.
3. Lack of signs of tissue necrosis anywhere in the body, or signs of inflammation in the cerebrospinal fluid.
4. Neurologic or pseudoneurologic symptoms in a majority of patients—apparently an excessive number compared to what is seen in systemic infectious diseases.
5. Primary myopathy, as judged by myalgic symptoms, possibly caused by the presence of viral genome in muscle (see Chapter 6).
6. Lack of mortality. Although many individuals with CFS are disabled, none die from the disorder; this is distinct from autoimmune diseases such as lupus erythematosus, multiple sclerosis, or myasthenic syndromes.

In reflecting on possible causes, we have developed certain interests which we would like to present in the hope that these ideas will stimulate work by others. Until CFS is less heterogeneous or until a specific biologic marker is developed, it seems to us that investigations of pathogenesis will be the best tactic.

Arguments Against Immunologic or Viral Mechanisms

Several explanations for the cause of CFS, which might appear to be plausible are increasingly unlikely. For instance, neurologists are quite accustomed to disease caused by immune assault on parts of the nervous system. Myasthenia gravis and Lambert-Eaton syndrome attack the neuromuscular junction, Guillain-Barré syndrome the peripheral nervous system, and multiple sclerosis the central nervous system, each with specificity. Several animal models are also well known. In all these instances, cell-mediated or antibody-mediated immunity can be demonstrated; in some, the disease can be passively transferred, and the antibody measured; or clinical improvement occurs with plasma exchange, with systemically administered immunoglobulin G (IgG), or with immunosuppression. By all these criteria, CFS is not immune mediated. As we pointed out, in autoimmune disease one expects a spectrum of illness, including a few fulminating and fatal cases, attesting to the potential power of the immune system. This is not observed in CFS.

Second, direct invasion of the nervous system by virus, at least by normal pathways, seems to us quite unlikely. In the past decade, interest in CFS was stimulated by several reports of an association between the disorder and elevated Epstein-Barr virus titers [13]. It now appears that this profile does not imply active virus infection but activation of antibody production associated with a separate, undefined illness. No other virus is currently a candidate to be a cause of CFS except for herpesvirus type 6, which has been associated with the recent Nevada epidemic [14]. Were this virus to be found causative, a novel means of disease production would have to be postulated.

Retrograde Transport of Viruses

The term *system disease* has been used to designate disorders of neurons that share a common pathologic vulnerability. Examples include highly selective pathologic changes that occur in motor neuron disease and spinocerebellar degenerations. One system of neurons that share a common vulnerability consists of all those which have endings outside the blood-brain barrier. No blood-to-nerve cell barrier exists in the circumventricular organs, the dorsal root ganglia, or any of the motor, sensory, or autonomic fibers that terminate outside the central nervous system. Certain toxins, viruses, neurotrophic factors, and various proteins and peptides may penetrate these terminals and may be transported to the cell bodies of origin via retrograde axoplasmic transport systems. For example, intravenously injected horseradish peroxidase (HRP) accumulates in the cell bodies of a variety of neurons via this mechanism [15].

These are the sites outside the blood-brain or blood-nerve barrier:

Dorsal root ganglion
Autonomic ganglia
Anterior horn cells
Cranial nerve homologues of the dorsal root and autonomic ganglia
The circumventricular organs (except the subfornical organ, where tight junctions exist in the capillaries):
  Median eminence
  Neurohypophysis
  Organosum vasculosum of the lamina terminalis
  Subcommisural organ
  Pineal gland
  Vertical limb of the diagonal band of Broca

Neurons in these sites that show retrograde labeling include the hypothalamic arcuate nucleus, the anterior periventricular stratum, and the supraoptic and paraventricular nuclei. HRP as a marker of retrograde transport is taken up at all types of terminals, but other molecules or viruses may show a high degree of specificity. Thus, there is a neural system driven by retrograde transport which is key to the pathogenesis of poliomyelitis, rabies, herpes zoster, labial and genital herpes, tetanus, and lead neuropathy [16–20]. After gaining access to the initial neuronal cell body in the central nervous system, a virus sequentially invades by specific transsynaptic spread with "amplification of the message'" at each subsequent neuron, and thus becomes widespread in the central nervous system without ever breaching the blood-brain barrier. This mechanism has been demonstrated in rabies, herpesvirus infections, and poliomyelitis [19,21,22].

In CFS, mixed disturbances of behavioral, motor, sensory, and autonomic function are seen. If the affected cells are injured but not killed, then the symptoms would fail to yield to our usual testing for neurologic deficits [23]. Recent studies in CFS have pointed to dysfunction of the hypothalamus [24,25], which might be especially vulnerable to retrograde transport. Mood changes, fatigue, sleep abnormalities, appetite changes, and altered temperature, vasomotor, and sleep regulation—which constitute 15 of the 29 most common symptoms listed for CFS [26]—could relate to disordered hypothalamic function.

Paresthesias and motor symptoms with unusual patterns might reflect retrograde invasion of sensory cells and lower motor neurons after invasion of distal processes. Deficits determined by retrograde transport may be in atypical distribution, and such novel factors as the amount of use may render a given body part more vulnerable to neurologic difficulties [20]. This occurs because turnover of the presynaptic membrane is proportional to the frequency of depolarization [27]: If toxins or viruses bind to the presynaptic membrane, then the dose accumulated in the neuronal cell body becomes proportional to the amount of synaptic activity of the most frequently used muscle. In the Bethesda epidemic, symptoms of weakness were much greater in the right arm than the left while lower extremity problems were equal [28].

Naturally, the deficits would not resemble the familiar neuropathic, myopathic, or central tract distributions, and therefore a functional label might result. This concept is not incompatible with the evidence of direct muscle involvement (see Chapter 9). Invasion of muscle along with retrograde motor and sensory nerves does occur in rabies, where the initial binding at acetylcholine receptor sites permits intramuscular proliferation of the virus during a prolonged latent phase. After this, the virus traverses the neuromuscular junction to penetrate the presynaptic membrane, ultimately becoming widespread within the nervous system through neuron-to-neuron transport [29].

Role of Cytokines

Cytokines might be involved in the production of CFS. Cytokines are soluble proteins secreted by cells. They are synthesized de novo after cell activation, and act on their target cells by binding to specific receptor sites with very high affinity. The majority have a molecular weight in the 15 to 25 kilodalton range, and for most of them the chromosomal location is known. Their presence can be detected in serum, and in some instances their solubilized receptors can be measured too. Cytokines can be classified as growth factors (interleukins 1–6), as activation factors (interferons), or as lymphotoxins (tumor necrosis factor [TNF], perforin). Typically, their effects are multiple and overlapping, and several factors will act synergistically or in a cascade in immune activation processes [30].

Interleukin-1 (IL-1) is a product of monocytes and macrophages. Binding of as few as 10 IL-1 receptors will activate a target cell [31], which is often a CD4 T cell. Increased IL-1 release is followed by a cascade of responses, including synthesis of interleukin-2 (IL-2), TNF, and cell adhesion molecules, and by maturation of B cells [31].

IL-1 has a number of nonimmunologic actions. Increased serum levels cause fever; apparently the cytokine enters the central nervous system through the lamina terminalis of the hypothalamus, which can be the locus of the febrile response. Neurons in this region may have IL-1 receptors [32] and can respond by releasing prostaglandin and eventually by stimulating production of adrenocorticotropic hormone (ACTH) [33].

Many conditions that cause proliferation of astrocytes, microglia, or macrophages may lead to increased concentrations of IL-1 in the brain, since all three cell types may be a source of IL-1 as well as of other cytokines [34]. Circulating IL-1 does not enter through an intact blood-brain barrier [30].

Tumor necrosis factor shows many stimulatory effects, often in synergy with IL-1. TNF receptors are found on many types of cells. The action of TNF often is to increase antigen presentation, to augment production of interferon-γ, and, with other cytokines, to cause proliferation of many cell types including endothelial cells. TNF has nonimmunologic activity. It was originally known as cachectin, since high levels are associated with weight loss, and it is also an endogenous pyrogen [30].

IL-2 is a product of activated T cells. It binds to other T cells, causing clonal expansion and further expression of additional cell types including B cells and NK cells as well as many other T-cell clones. For example, serum IL-2 levels are elevated in patients with active multiple sclerosis, reflecting the presence of activated T cells in the circulation [35]. Similarly, there may be an elevation of soluble IL-2α receptors (recognized by Tac), and an increased number of Tac-positive reactive cells can be thought of as a measure of an activated immune response [36]. Both serum and CSF levels of cytokines can be measured in multiple sclerosis [34,37] and could be assessed in CFS as well.

IL-2 has striking nonimmunologic effects. It is now widely used on an experimental basis for treatment of some advanced malignancies [38]. After systemic administration at high doses, patients experience malaise, fatigue, fever, myalgia, and fluid retention. A vascular leak syndrome with edema and hypotension has been observed [38]. The myalgia [39] may be a reflection of proteolysis [40]. IL-2 may have neuropsychiatric effects [41]. Typically, these will begin on the fourth or fifth day of treatment even though it is known that the protein enters the cerebrospinal fluid rapidly and more completely than would be predicted by its size [42]. The neuropsychiatric symptoms include disorientation, hallucinations, and even coma. Except for fatigue, all the side effects of IL-2 administration are markedly reduced at low doses [43]. Possibly the neurologic effects of IL-2 administered systemically require uptake by nerve terminals in the manner we have described. A few preliminary measurements of cytokine levels in cerebrospinal fluid, apparently inconclusive, have been made [44–46].

A number of other cytokines are known; it is beyond the scope of this chapter to list all of them. Inhibitory molecules might be relevant to CFS (or to the cessation of CFS). Transforming growth factor (TGFβ) is one of these. It often acts late in an immune response to reduce proliferation of induced T and B cells [30]. For instance, administration of TGFβ can block experimental allergic encephalomyelitis in rats [47]. Interleukin-6 can be inhibitory in some circumstances.

Cytokines may be involved in central nervous system function in unexpected ways. They may be regulated by hormones; for instance, melanocyte-stimulating hormone (an analog of ACTH) may regulate levels of TNF and of inducible IL-1 biologic responses [33]; we are accustomed to ACTH release from the hypothalamic-pituitary axis as a source for steroid responses from the adrenal gland, but there may be immunologic effects too.

Measurement of serum and cerebrospinal fluid levels of relevant cytokines may be a fruitful approach to CFS. Control data will be critical. Levels of cytokines are known to change with either bacterial [48] or viral meningitis [49], and of course an interferon response to any viral infection is to be expected.

OBSERVATIONS ABOUT THERAPY

Are there any lessons thus far from therapeutic trials in CFS? On the whole we would say no. Of antiviral agents, only acyclovir has been rigorously tested, with negative results [50]. The symptomatic treatments reviewed in Chapter 14 give no etiologic clues. Efforts to immunosuppress have been fruitless. Two trials with intravenous IgG are known to us; a U.S. trial gave negative results [51], while an Australian trial, with a larger dose, showed a positive effect [52]. A recent trial of an unsaturated fatty acid preparation was blinded and showed clear benefit [53]. This result is of interest since it is known that administration of n-3 unsaturated fatty acids can reduce the synthesis of IL-1 and TNF by mononuclear cells [54]. This trial needs to be repeated by other investigators since it appears to provide a definite lead.

In a disease with no clear clinical definition, no accepted laboratory guidelines, a substantial spontaneous remission rate, and a large placebo response rate [50], adherence to well-designed placebo-controlled prospective trials of any potential therapy seems mandatory. In the meantime, one can only hope that disabled patients and their health care providers, whether they follow a traditional or alternative style of practice, will be tolerant of the medical efforts to define this baffling illness further.

REFERENCES

1. Shorter, E. *From Paralysis to Fatigue: A History of Psychosomatic Illness in the Modern Era.* New York: Free Press, 1991.
2. Wessely, S. Myalgic encephalomyelitis—A warning: Discussion paper. *J. R. Soc. Med.* 82:215, 1989.
3. Chen, M. The epidemiology of self-perceived fatigue among adults. *Prevent. Med.* 15:74, 1986.
4. Manu, P., Lane, T.J., and Matthews, D.A. The frequency of the chronic

fatigue syndrome in patients with symptoms of persistent fatigue. *Ann. Intern. Med.* 109:554, 1988.

5. Buchwald, D., and Komaroff, A.L. Review of laboratory findings for patients with chronic fatigue syndrome. *Rev. Infect. Dis.* 13 (Suppl. 1):S12, 1991.

6. Buchwald, D., Cheney, P.R., Peterson, D.L., et al. A chronic illness characterized by fatigue, neurologic and immunologic disorders, and active human herpes virus type 6 infection. *Ann. Intern. Med.* 11:102, 1992.

7. Landry, A.L., Jessop, C., Lennette, E.T., et al. Chronic fatigue syndrome: Clinical condition associated with immune activation. *Lancet* 338:707, 1991.

8. Lloyd, A.R., Wakefield, D., Broughton, L.R., et al. Immunologic abnormalities in the chronic fatigue syndrome. *Med. J. Aust.* 151:122, 1989.

9. DeFreitas, E., Hilliard, B., Cheney, P.R., et al. Retroviral sequences related to human T-lymphotrophic virus type II in patients with chronic fatigue immune dysfunction syndrome. *Proc. Natl. Acad. Sci. USA* 88:2922, 1991.

10. Shafran, S.D. The chronic fatigue syndrome. *Am. J. Med.* 90:730, 1991.

11. Byrne, E., and Trounce, I. Chronic fatigue and myalgia syndrome: Mitochondrial and glycolytic studies in skeletal muscle. *J. Neurol. Neurosurg. Psychiatry* 50:743, 1987.

12. Lane, T.J., Mathews, D.A., and Manu, P. The low yield of physical examinations and laboratory investigations of patients with chronic fatigue. *Am. J. Med. Sci.* 299:313, 1990.

13. Strauss, S.E., Tosato, G., Armstrong, G., et al. Persisting illness and fatigue in adults with evidence of Epstein-Barr virus infection. *Ann. Intern. Med.* 102:7, 1985.

14. Daugherty, S.A., Henry, B.E., Peterson, D.L., et al. Chronic fatigue syndrome in northern Nevada. *Rev. Infect. Dis.* 13 (Suppl. 1):S39, 1991.

15. Broadwell, R.D., and Brightman, M.W. Entry of peroxidase into neurons of the central and peripheral nervous systems from extracerebral and cerebral blood. *J. Comp. Neurol.* 166:257, 1976.

16. Brown, R.H., Jr., Johnson, D., Ogonowsk, R.A., and Weiner, H.L. Type 1 human poliovirus binds to human synaptosomes. *Ann. Neurol.* 21:64, 1987.

17. Fishman, P.S., and Carrigan, D.R. Motoneuron uptake from the circulation of the binding fragment of tetanus toxin. *Arch. Neurol.* 45:558, 1988.

18. Nahmias, A.J., and Roizman, B. Infection with herpes-simplex viruses 1 and 2. *N. Engl. J. Med.* 289:667, 1973.

19. Rupprecht, C.E., and Dietzschold, B. Perspectives on rabies virus pathogenesis. *Lab. Invest.* 57:603, 1987.

20. Sabin, T.D. Classification of peripheral neuropathy: The long and the short of it. *Muscle Nerve* 9:711, 1986.

21. Jubelt, B., Narayan, O., and Johnson, R.T. Pathogenesis of human poliovirus infection in mice. *J. Neuropathol. Exp. Neurol.* 39:149, 1980.

22. Ugolini, G., Kuypers, H.G.J.M., and Strick, P.L. Transneuronal transfer of herpes-virus from peripheral nerves to cortex and brainstem. *Science* 243:89, 1989.

23. Southern, P., and Oldstone, M.B.A. Medical consequences of persistent viral infection. *N. Engl. J. Med.* 314:359, 1986.

24. Behan, P.O., and Bokhett, A.M.O. Clinical spectrum of postviral fatigue syndrome. *Br. Med. Bull.* 47:793, 1991.

25. Demitrack, M.A. Evidence for impaired activation of the hypothalamic-pituitary-adrenal axis in patients with chronic fatigue syndrome. *J. Clin. Endocrinol. Metab.* 73:1224, 1991.

26. Holmes, G.P., Kaplan, J.E., Gantz, N.M., et al. Chronic fatigue syndrome: A working case definition. *Ann. Intern. Med.* 108:387, 1988.

27. Heuser, J.E., and Reese, T.S. Evidence for recycling of synaptic vesicle mem-

brane during transmitter release at the frog neuromuscular junction. *J. Cell. Biol.* 57:315, 1973.

28. Shelokov, A., Habel, K., Verder, E., et al. Epidemic neuromyasthenia. *N. Engl. J. Med.* 257:345, 1957.

29. Lentz, T.L., Wilson, P.T., Hawrot, E., et al. Amino acid sequence similarity between rabies virus glycoprotein and snake venom curaremimetic neurotoxins. *Science* 226:847, 1984.

30. Arnason, B.G.W., and Reder, R.T. Cell mediated immunity and neurologic disease. In A.K. Asbury, G.M. McKhann, and W.I. McDonald (eds.). *Diseases of the Nervous System: Clinical Neurobiology* (2nd ed.). Philadelphia: Saunders, 1992.

31. Dinarello, C.A. Interleukin-1 and its biologically related cytokines. *Adv. Immunol.* 44:153, 1989.

32. Breder, L.D., Dinarello, C.A., and Saper, C.B. Interleukin-1 immunoreactive innervation of the human hypothalamus. *Science* 240:321, 1988.

33. Robertson, B., Dostal, K., and Dagnes, R.A. Neuropeptide regulation of inflammatory and immunologic responses: The capacity of alpha-melanocyte stimulating hormone to inhibit tumor necrosis factor and IL-1 inducible biologic responses. *J. Immunol.* 140:4300, 1988.

34. Hauser, S.L., Doolittle, T.H., Lincoln, R., et al. Cytokine accumulations in the CSF of multiple sclerosis patients: Frequent detection of interleukin-1 and tumor necrosis factor but not interleukin-6. *Neurology* 40:1735, 1990.

35. Bellamy, A.S., Calder, V.L., Feldmann, M., et al. The distribution of interleukin-2 receptor bearing lymphocytes in multiple sclerosis: Evidence for a key role of activated lymphocytes. *Clin. Exp. Immunol.* 61:248, 1985.

36. Adachi, K., Kumamoto, T., Araki, S. Elevated soluble interleukin-2 receptor levels in patients with active multiple sclerosis. *Ann. Neurol.* 28:687, 1990.

37. Gallo, P., Piccinno, M.G., Pagni, S., et al. Immune activation in multiple sclerosis: Study of IL-2, SIL-2R and gamma-IFN levels in serum and cerebrospinal fluid. *J. Neurol. Sci.* 92:9, 1989.

38. Hamblin, T.J. Interleukin-2. *Br. Med. J.* 300:275, 1990.

39. Wallace, D.J., Margolin, K., and Waller, P. Fibromyalgia and interleukin-2 therapy for malignancy. *Ann. Intern. Med.* 108:909, 1988.

40. Baracos, V., Rodemann, H.P., Dinarello, C.A., et al. Stimulation of muscle protein degradation and prostaglandin E_2 release by leukocytic pyrogen (interleukin-1): A mechanism for the increased degradation of muscle protein during fever. *N. Engl. J. Med.* 308:553, 1983.

41. Denicoff, K.D., Rubinow, D.R., and Pape, M.S. The neuropsychiatric effects of treatment with interleukin-2 and lymphokine activated killer cells. *Ann. Intern. Med.* 84:1072, 1987.

42. Saris, S.C., Rosenberg, S.A., Friedman, R.B., et al. Penetration of recombinant interleukin-2 across the blood cerebrospinal fluid barrier. *J. Neurosurg.* 69:29, 1988.

43. Soiffer, R.J., Murray, C., Cochran, K., et al. Clinical and immunologic effects of prolonged infusion of low dose recombinant interleukin-2 after autologous and T-cell-depleted allogenic bone marrow transplantation. *Blood* 79:517, 1992.

44. Cheney, P.R., Dorman, S.E., and Bell, D.S. Interleukin-2 and the chronic fatigue syndrome [letter]. *Ann. Intern. Med.* 110:321, 1989.

45. Lever, A.M.L., Lewis, D.M., Bwennister, B.A., et al. Interferon production in postviral fatigue syndrome [letter]. *Lancet* 2:101, 1988.

46. Strauss, S.E., Dale, J.K., Peter, J.B., et al. Circulating lymphokine levels in the chronic fatigue syndrome. *J. Infect. Dis.* 160:1085, 1989.

47. Schleuscher, H.J. Transforming growth factors type beta$_1$ and beta$_2$ suppress

rat astrocyte autoantigen presentation and antagonize hyperinduction of class II major histocompatibility complex antigen expression by interferon gamma and tumor necrosis factor. *J. Neuroimmunol.* 27:41, 1990.

48. Mustafa, M., Mertsola, J., Ramilo, O., et al. Increased endotoxin and interleukin-1 concentrations in cerebrospinal fluid of infants with coliform meningitis and ventriculitis associated with intraventricular gentamicin therapy. *J. Infect. Dis.* 160:891, 1989.

49. Frei, K., Leist, T.P., Meager, A., et al. Production of B cell stimulatory factor-2 and interferon gamma in the central nervous system during viral meningitis and encephalitis. *J. Exp. Med.* 168:449, 1988.

50. Strauss, S.E., Dale, J.K., Tobi, M., et al. Acyclovir treatment of the chronic fatigue syndrome: Lack of efficacy in a placebo-controlled trial. *N. Engl. J. Med.* 319:1692, 1988.

51. Peterson, P.K., Shepard, J., Macres, M., et al. A controlled trial of intravenous IgG in chronic fatigue syndrome. *Am. J. Med.* 89:554, 1990.

52. Lloyd, A., Hickie, I., Wakefield, D., et al. A double-blind, placebo-controlled trial of intravenous immunoglobulin therapy in patients with chronic fatigue syndrome. *Am. J. Med.* 89:561, 1990.

53. Behan, P.O., and Behan, W.M.H. Essential fatty acids in the treatment of postviral fatigue syndrome. In D.F. Horrobin (ed.). *Omega-6 Essential Fatty Acids: Pathophysiology and Roles in Clinical Medicine.* New York: Wiley-Liss, 1990.

54. Endres, S., Ghorbani, B.S., Kelley, V.F., et al. The effect of dietary supplementation with n-3 polyunsaturated fatty acids on the synthesis of interleukin-1 and tumor necrosis factor by mononuclear cells. *N. Engl. J. Med.* 5:265, 1989.

Index